The Grisly History of Medicine
Killer Bugs

Written by John Farndon
Illustrated by Venitia Dean

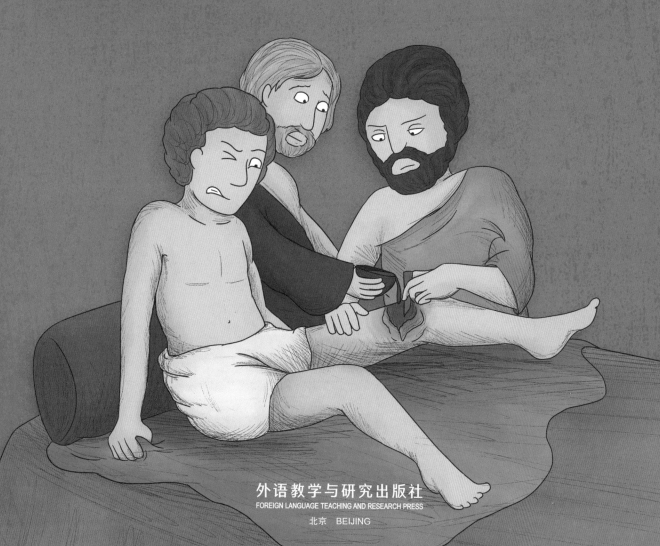

外语教学与研究出版社
FOREIGN LANGUAGE TEACHING AND RESEARCH PRESS
北京　BEIJING

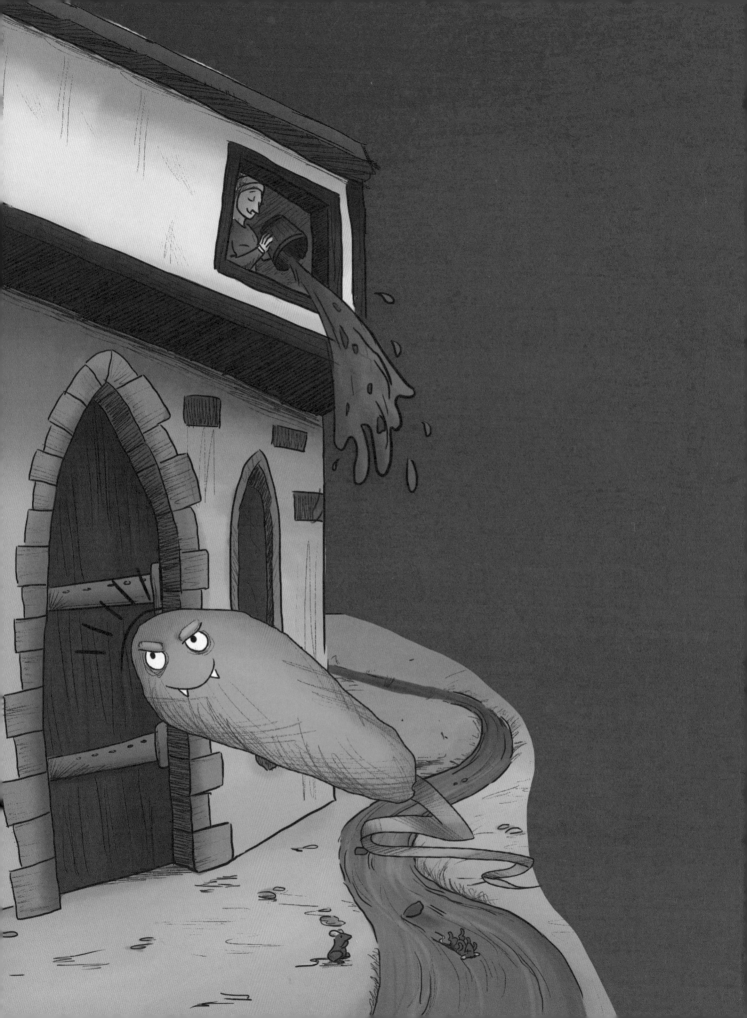

Invisible microbes cause sickness by setting up home in our bodies and multiplying – fast! Follow the hunt for these tiny killers over thousands of years, and the fight to outwit and eliminate them.

- Smallpox and tuberculosis came from cattle
- Cholera made the skin shrivel and turn blue
- Hospitals caused fatal diseases

...

Find out how the French scientist Louis Pasteur unmasked germs living in the air, the German doctor Robert Koch proved that they caused disease, and the British surgeon Joseph Lister pioneered surgery in super-clean conditions – some of the greatest victories in the battle against disease.

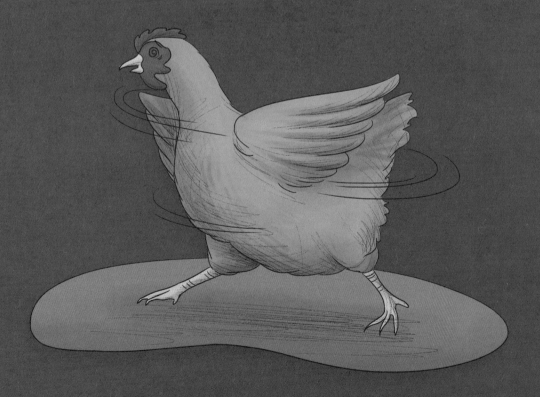

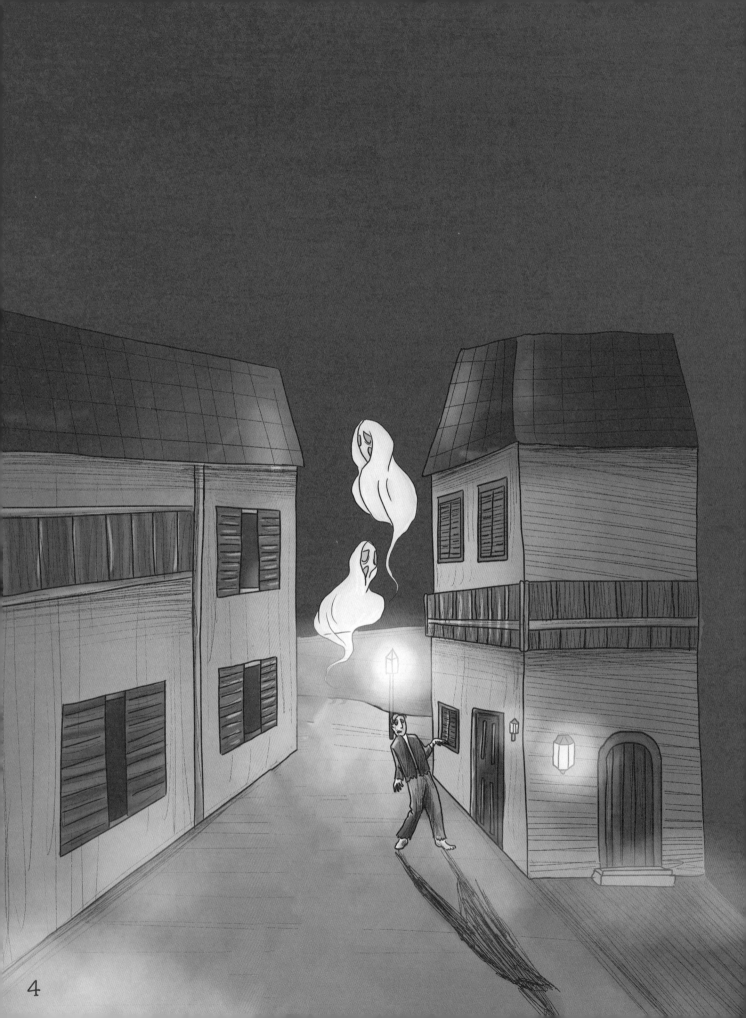

Contents

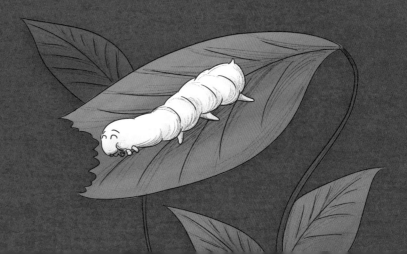

INTRODUCTION

Germs are tiny organisms that make you sick. Because they're far too small to see, they sneak into your body without you noticing and then infect you with all kinds of terrible diseases.
This book tells the story of how these tiny monsters were finally unmasked...

Home wreckers

Germs don't actually try to make us ill. It's just that bodies like ours make very good homes for them, and once they get inside, they multiply rapidly to make the most of their good luck! That's how they do the damage.

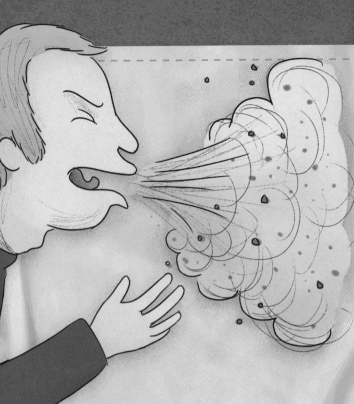

Catching germs

Germs are found all over the world, in all kinds of places. Some reach you through the air via sneezes, coughs or someone's breath. You can also become infected if you touch somewhere contaminated with germs, then touch your nose and breathe in. Other germs can be swallowed when you eat bad food.

Defenders

Luckily, your body has an amazing defence system for dealing with germs called the 'immune system'. It's a complex army of tiny cells that circulate in your blood and do battle with germs. It often takes time to kick in, though. That's why you get ill – then, with luck, recover because your immune system has dealt with them.

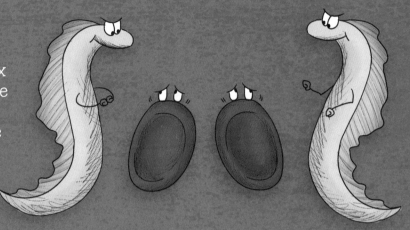

Doctor's orders

Doctors have two ways of helping your body fight germs. One is with vaccination, which primes your body's immune system to fight particular germs. The other is with antibiotics – chemicals that you usually swallow in pills – which are poisonous to germs.

Keeping clean

There's another way we can reduce the danger of germs – by cleanliness, or 'hygiene'. Many germs spread in dirt, so by keeping things clean we reduce the chances of infection. That's why it's good to wash your hands.

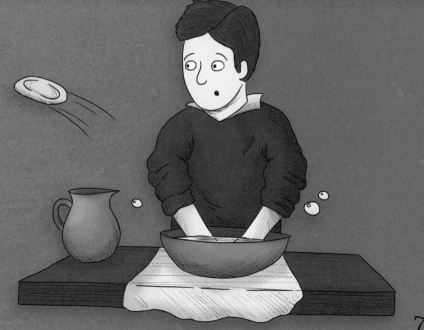

SETTLING FOR GERMS

In the early days of mankind, when people roamed around hunting and gathering, infectious diseases were probably rare. People did not live close enough together for germs to spread, or stay long enough near water sources to pollute them.

Disease on the farm

The development of farming some 10,000 years ago saved mankind from starvation and provided food for the first towns and cities. But we now know that germs multiplied as people and farm animals began living close together, sharing their germs, and water became polluted.

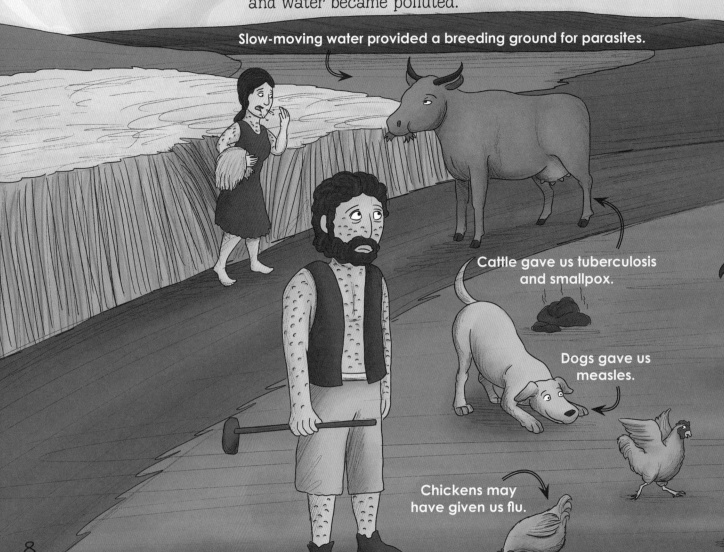

Slow-moving water provided a breeding ground for parasites.

Cattle gave us tuberculosis and smallpox.

Dogs gave us measles.

Chickens may have given us flu.

The first known polio victim?

On an Egyptian stele from over 3,000 years ago, there is a picture of a man using a cane for support. He seems to have a withered leg, which could be caused by polio. If so, he is the first known victim of this terrible disease, which may have developed in water dirtied by the dung of farm animals.

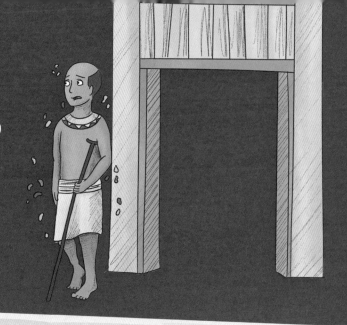

As farming became more intense, manure-polluted water encouraged diseases such as polio, cholera, typhoid and hepatitis. Slow-moving irrigation water provided ideal conditions for parasites such as those causing the diseases bilharzia and malaria.

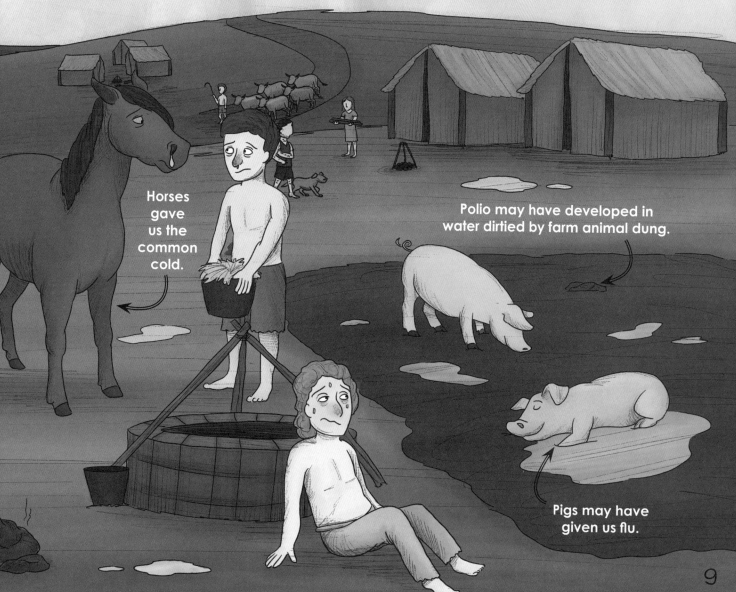

Horses gave us the common cold.

Polio may have developed in water dirtied by farm animal dung.

Pigs may have given us flu.

BAD AIR

Few people had any idea diseases were spread by tiny invisible germs. Most thought bad, smelly air was to blame – especially damp, misty air near ditches and swamps. This nasty mist was called a 'miasma'.

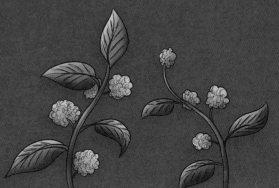

Dealing with odours

Most people in ancient India, as elsewhere in the world, thought disease was caused by poisonous air. They chewed a paste made from the leaves of the gambir tree as an antidote.

Morning smells

The Roman writer Vitruvius was convinced it was a very bad idea to build a city anywhere near swamps. He believed morning breezes would blow miasmas from the marshes, along with the poisonous breath of swamp creatures, to the city and make people ill.

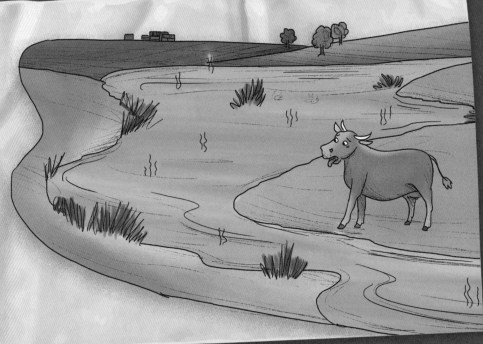

Taking it in the South

Government officials in ancient China knew they were in trouble if they were sent off to the mountainous regions in the South! Because it was usually damp and misty there, and people were convinced that poisonous air would make them fall ill and die.

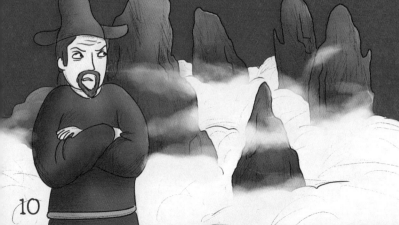

Evil mist in New Orleans

The city of New Orleans often suffered from outbreaks of disease. People were convinced this was because of bad air full of evil spirits coming from the nearby swamps. So they burned huge bonfires of feverfew plants and fired cannons into the swamps to keep the evil mist at bay.

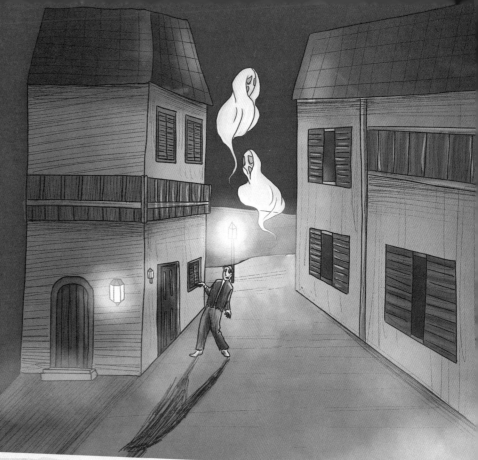

Taking drinking water from the river could be fatal.

The Great Stink

In the past, so much sewage poured into the River Thames in London that in the hot summer of 1858, the stink coming off it was bad enough to make you throw up. They called it the Great Stink and people began to leave the city – convinced the terrible smell of sewage gas caused deadly disease. To solve the problem, London built the first modern sewerage system.

11

EASTERN IDEAS

You might think people had no idea about germs in the past because they are just too small to see. But in India thousands of years ago, those who followed Jainism were taught that tiny life forms called 'nigodas' existed all around them.

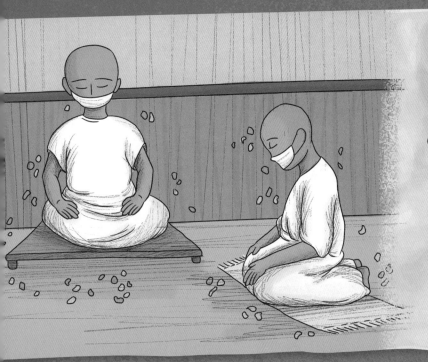

Saving germs

Just as people nowadays often wear surgical masks in order not to breathe in germs, so did the Jains, thousands of years ago. But their aim was not to avoid disease. They believed they must not harm any living thing, and wanted to avoid killing the tiny nigodas by accidentally swallowing them!

Ancient medicine

Ayurveda is an ancient medical system, developed in India more than 3,000 years ago, that uses complex mixes of herbs to treat people. Scientists are not sure if it works, but many people still use it. Ayurvedists believed that microbes caused diseases such as leprosy and meningitis.

Prevention better than cure

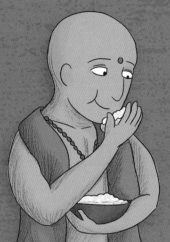

One of the most important old texts of Ayurvedic medicine was the *Charaka-Samhita*, edited about 2,000 years ago by Charaka. According to the text, prevention is better than cure. That's why different diets were suggested to keep people healthy in different places and at different times of year.

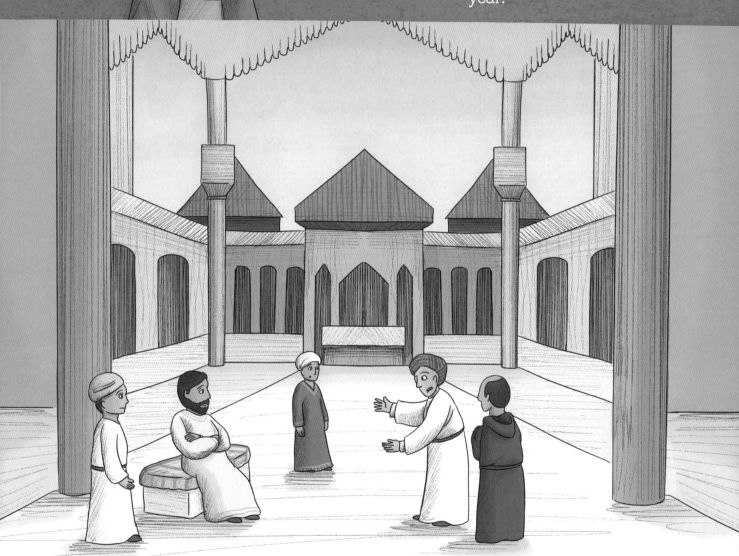

The plague in Granada

Around 1350, the bubonic plague reached Granada in Spain, then part of the Islamic world. Physician Ibn Khatima suggested it was spread by 'minute bodies', which sound rather like germs. Another physician, al-Khatib – shown in the orange headscarf with a high-ranking official in Granada's Alhambra Palace – explained how such 'minute bodies' spread the plague by contact between people.

INVISIBLE ANIMALS

Around 1590, Dutch spectacle maker Zacharias Jansen put some lenses together – and invented the microscope. When people began to look through it, they were blown away by what they saw: a whole new unknown world of tiny organisms, too small to see normally.

Hooked in

In 1665, the English physicist Robert Hooke (1635–1703) published *Micrographia*, a book full of drawings of the amazing things he viewed down a microscope – things people had never seen before. In slices of cork, he could see a honeycomb network of boxes. He called the boxes 'cells', and we now know all living things are built up from tiny cells.

Tiny monsters

Dutch scientist Anton van Leeuwenhoek (1632–1723) made a microscope with just a single lens. It was simple but brilliant, and he could see things 200 times larger than life! He discovered that clear water is not clear at all, but teeming with tiny creatures. In fact, there are tiny creatures almost everywhere.

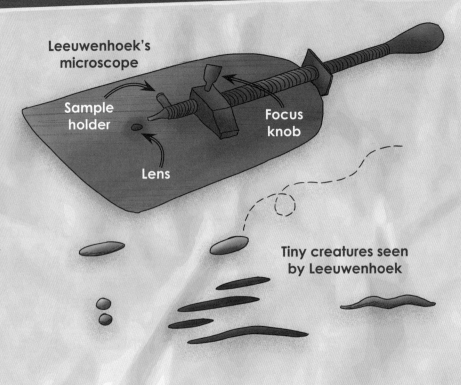

Leeuwenhoek's microscope

Sample holder

Focus knob

Lens

Tiny creatures seen by Leeuwenhoek

14

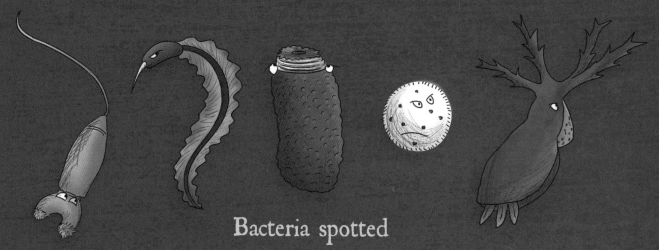

Bacteria spotted

Leeuwenhoek was astonished by the range of creatures he saw (above). Many looked like monsters. It was Leeuwenhoek who saw bacteria for the first time. When he looked through his microscope at plaque taken from human teeth, he saw bacteria wriggling in it.

The bacteria four

After Leeuwenhoek's great discovery, no one paid much attention to bacteria for the next 200 years, until German biologist Ferdinand Cohn began to study them closely in the 1870s. Cohn realised that, though there were many kinds of bacteria, they could be divided into four groups, depending on their shapes: spheres, rods, threads and spirals.

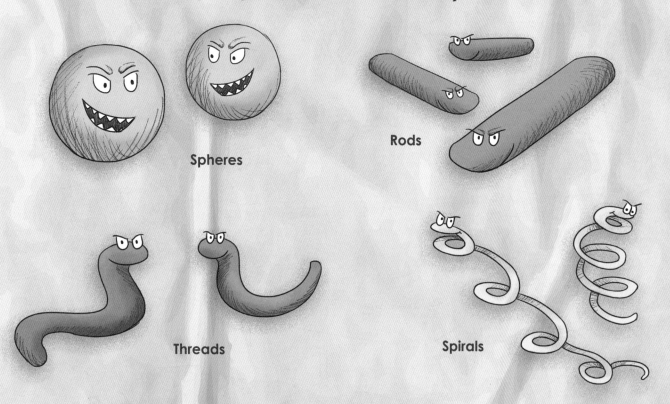

Spheres

Rods

Threads

Spirals

NOW WASH YOUR HANDS

Hospitals in the past were deadly dangerous! Very few people knew that germs caused disease, so doctors and nurses spread disease as they went from patient to patient, with terrible consequences.

Don't take me to the hospital!

Giving birth at home was never easy for young mums. But hospitals were deadly. Doctors carried the killer childbed or 'puerperal' fever on their hands, and spread it from one young mum to the next. So going into hospital to give birth could be a death sentence!

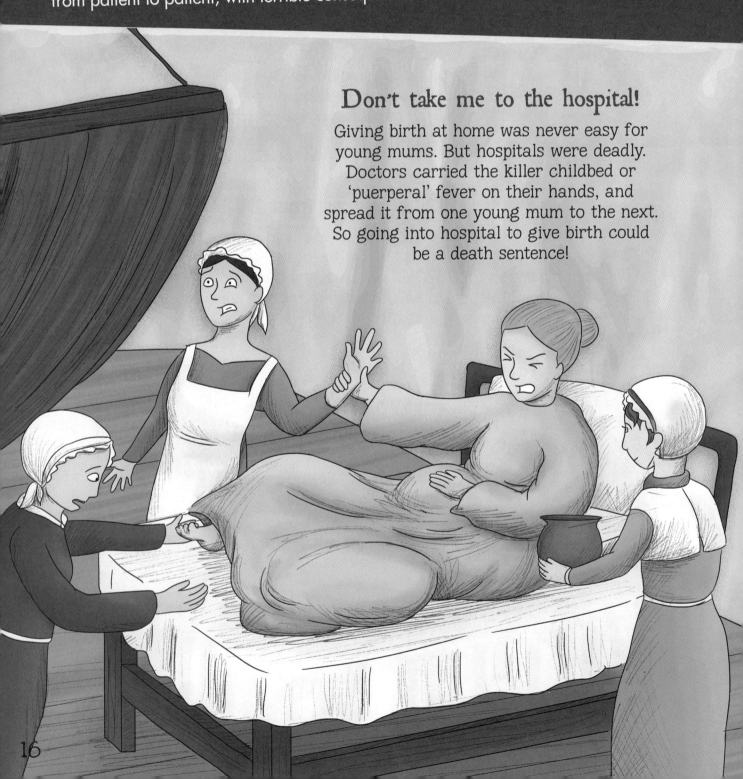

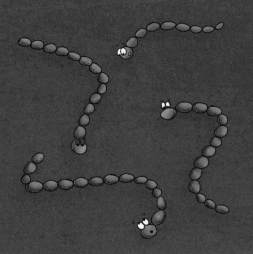

The real culprit

Of course, the doctors weren't really to blame. Their unwashed hands were simply carrying the germs that were the real culprits. As we now know, the germ that causes childbed fever is the bacterium *Streptococcus pyogenes*. Fortunately, proper hygiene in hospitals means this germ very rarely has its evil way!

Trust me, I'm a doctor!

In Vienna General Hospital in the 1800s, doctors often handled diseased corpses in the mortuary, then nipped next door to Maternity Ward 1 to examine mums-to-be – with fatal results. When the young Hungarian doctor Ignaz Semmelweis (1818–1865) arrived in 1847, he was appalled by the high death rate on the ward – and realised the doctors were to blame.

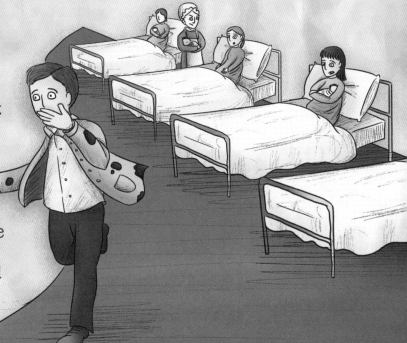

My hands are clean

Semmelweis ordered all medical staff to wash their hands regularly in calcium chloride. At once, death rates on Maternity Ward 1 dropped. But doctors could not believe they were to blame. They sacked Semmelweis, and carried on as before. It was a while before everyone realised just how important cleanliness, or 'hygiene', is in stopping germs spreading.

DIRTY DRAINS

In the 1800s, London and other European cities grew rapidly – and so did deaths from the killer disease cholera. Poor people were especially hard hit by cholera.

Feeling blue

Cholera is a horrible disease that seems to have originated in India on the banks of the Ganges River. Victims may suffer from diarrhoea so severe that their bodies are drained of water. Their eyes go hollow, their skin shrivels and they turn blue.

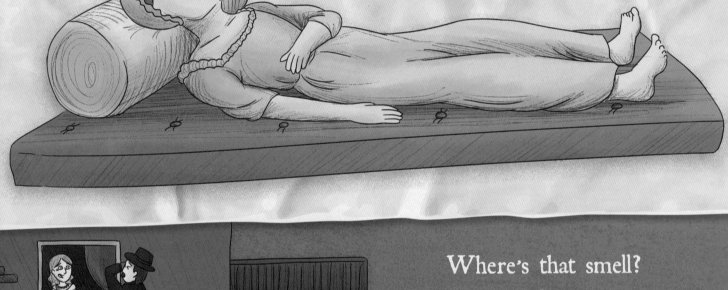

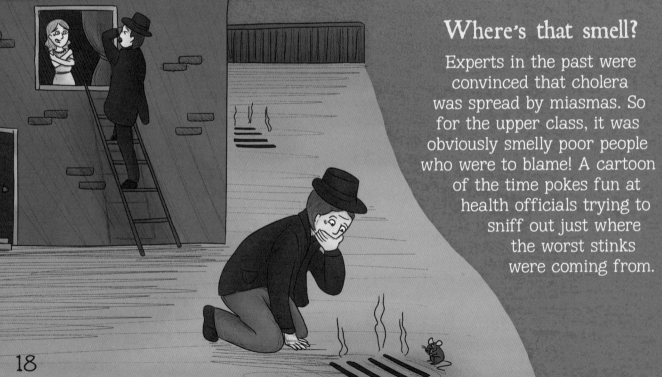

Where's that smell?

Experts in the past were convinced that cholera was spread by miasmas. So for the upper class, it was obviously smelly poor people who were to blame! A cartoon of the time pokes fun at health officials trying to sniff out just where the worst stinks were coming from.

The Soho pump

English doctor John Snow didn't think the miasma theory was right. When cholera hit London's Soho district in 1854, he found that all the victims had drunk water from just one pump in Broadwick Street. Human poo had contaminated the water supply for the pump. But it was a while before people understood that cholera is caused by germs in dirty water.

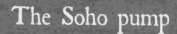

The fast way to travel

The opening of Egypt's Suez Canal in 1869 cut the sea journey from India to Europe dramatically – and made it much easier for cholera epidemics to spread. London escaped the worst because by then it had built good sewers, but many other European cities suffered badly.

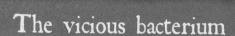

The vicious bacterium

In 1854, cholera hit Florence in Italy, the same year that it hit London's Soho. In Florence, microbiologist Filippo Pacini looked down his microscope and identified the culprit: the bacterium *Vibrio cholerae*. But everyone ignored him, since they thought miasmas were to blame. Then in 1883, German doctor Robert Koch (1843–1910), too, nailed *Vibrio cholerae* as the cause of cholera – and he was so famous that everyone believed him!

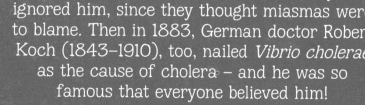

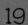

GUILTY GERMS

In the 1840s and 1850s, Semmelweis and Snow showed how clean hands and good drains could cut the spread of disease. So how could bad air be to blame? Then in the 1860s, the French microbiologist Louis Pasteur (1822–1895) began to demonstrate that the real culprits are microbes.

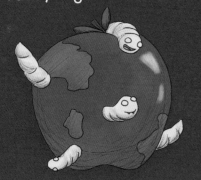

Life from nothing

When people saw maggots crawling from rotten apples or dead meat, it didn't occur to them the maggots had hatched from eggs. They thought they simply appeared whenever food rotted. This idea of life appearing from nothing is known as 'spontaneous generation'.

Life from the air

In 1859, Pasteur demonstrated with a simple experiment that microbes won't appear magically by spontaneous generation when food decays. Instead, they fall from the air on dust.

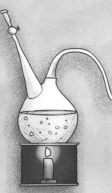

1. Pasteur boiled meat broth in a flask with a bent 'swan' neck to kill off any microbes.

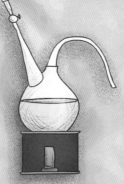

2. The swan neck stopped dust falling in, so the broth stayed clear.

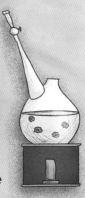

3. He then broke off the neck to allow dust to fall in. The broth quickly went cloudy, showing microbes were multiplying.

Microbes on worms

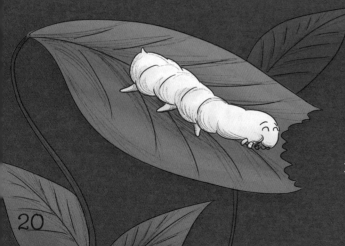

In 1867, Pasteur showed that microbes can cause disease. He had been studying a disease that was killing silkworms. When Pasteur examined the diseased worms through his microscope, he found they were infected by not just one kind of microbe, but two.

Chicken experiment

In 1879, Pasteur discovered how to protect people against germs with experiments on chickens. He grew chicken cholera germs in a dish, then starved them of nutrition so they became weak. When he injected chickens with these weakened germs, the chickens became immune to the disease. Vaccinating people with weakened germs is now one of the main ways of preventing diseases.

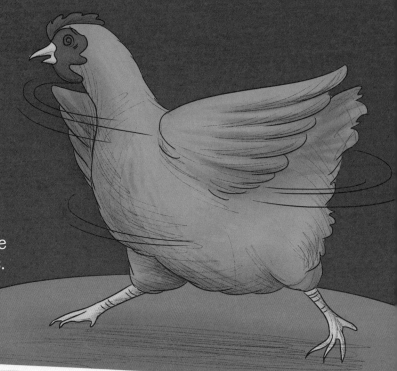

Sheep shot

In 1881, Pasteur also found a way to weaken the germs that cause anthrax in sheep. Using these weakened germs, he vaccinated sheep so that they became immune to anthrax.

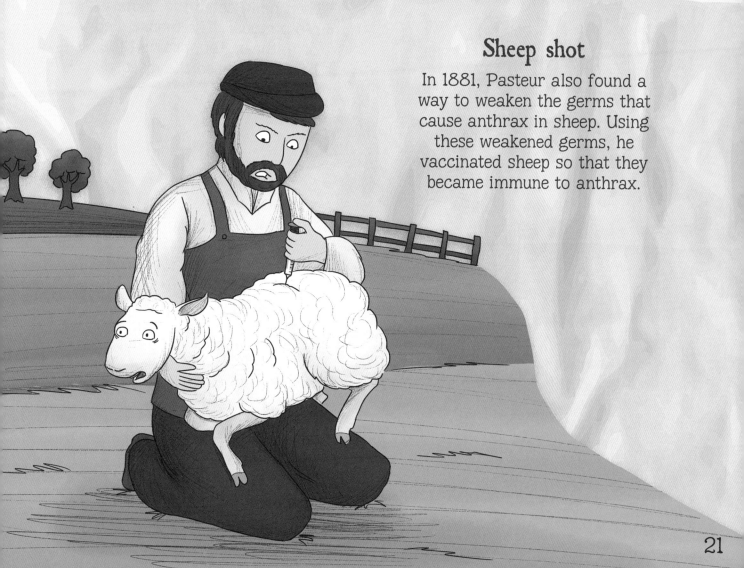

GERMS NAILED

Louis Pasteur proved there are microbes in the air, and that they can cause disease. Then Robert Koch showed there's a whole army of nasty microbes out there – and that it's these nasty microbes that are to blame for most diseases.

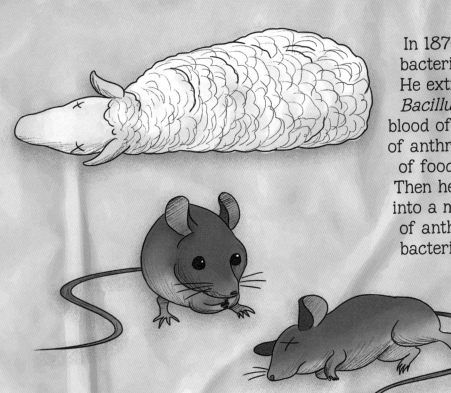

Guilty!

In 1876, Koch proved that bacteria can cause disease. He extracted the bacterium *Bacillus anthracis* from the blood of a sheep that had died of anthrax and put it in a dish of food so that it multiplied. Then he injected the bacteria into a mouse. The mouse died of anthrax, too, proving the bacteria caused the disease.

The criminal

Bacillus anthracis is a rod-shaped organism. It's so tiny you can only see it under a microscope. But despite its small size, it can kill a sheep or even a person. It does its damage by multiplying dramatically in the body and releasing a poison.

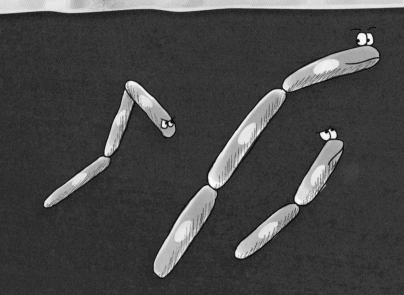

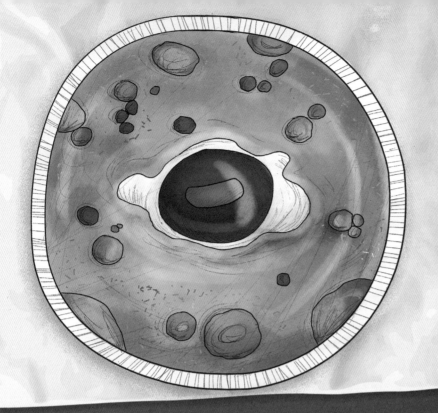

Cultured germs

Koch's work with germs depended on growing them in a dish in the laboratory. Growths like this are called 'cultures', and they need food. At first, Koch used the liquid from an ox's eye as food for germ cultures. Later he developed a broth of agar (a jelly made from algae) and gelatine (a jelly made from animal bones).

Koch's postulates: the four tests

Koch's work led him to establish four tests for proving which germ causes a disease.

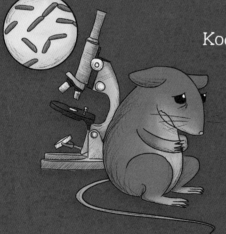

1. Association: the germ and the disease are seen together all the time.

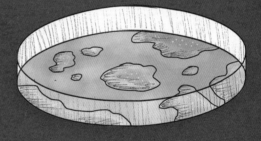

2. Isolation: the germ can be taken from the diseased animal and grown as a pure culture.

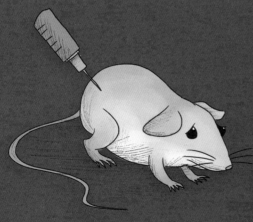

3. Inoculation: the germ taken from the diseased animal causes the disease in a healthy animal.

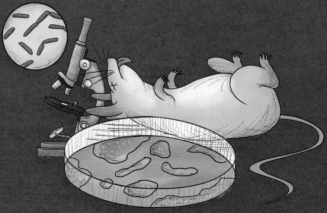

4. Re-isolation: the germ can also be taken from the newly infected animal.

23

CLEAN SURGERY

If germs cause disease, how do we stop them? One answer is to keep clean. Semmelweis showed how important it was to keep clean when mothers gave birth. British surgeon Joseph Lister (1827–1912) showed how vital it was for surgery.

Mummy, you're rotten

Dead bodies rot away because they are attacked by microbes. But the Ancient Egyptians learnt how to stop the rot by turning the bodies into mummies. This meant soaking the body in 'embalming fluids' that were poisonous to microbes.

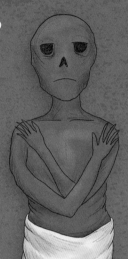

Pus is bad

The 13th-century surgeon Hugh of Lucca realised the danger of wounds becoming infected and so he cleaned them with wine. He knew that pus oozing from a wound was a bad sign, showing the wound was infected. Most doctors at the time thought (wrongly) that pus was a sign that the wound was getting better.

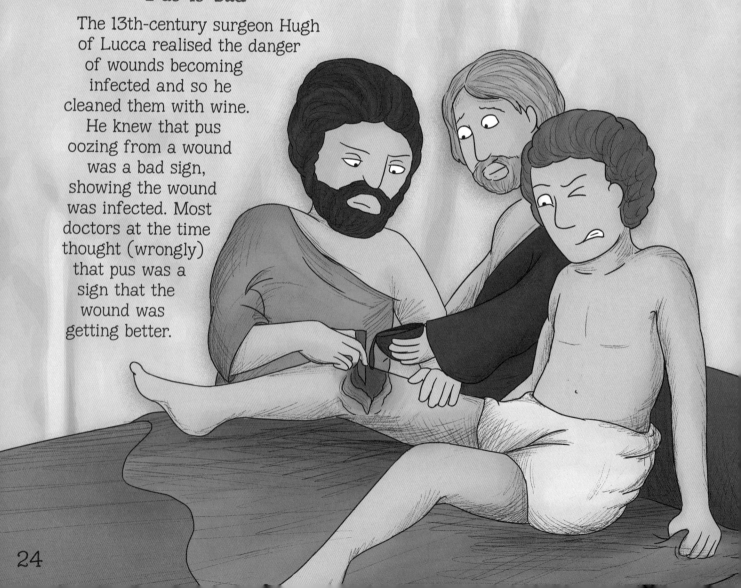

Filth

The growing cities of the 1800s were filthy places, because they had no proper rubbish collection, a poor water supply and a lack of good drains. In such conditions, germs could spread easily. Hospitals were among the worst culprits for germ-friendly filth!

Clean surgery

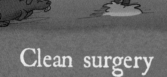

Until the 1860s, all too many patients undergoing surgery died of infections afterwards. Then Joseph Lister introduced the idea of 'antiseptic' surgery. He made sure that hands, instruments and surfaces were thoroughly washed with germ-killing chemicals such as carbolic soap. The idea worked, and now it is standard practice around the world.

Masked doctors

Lister's antiseptic methods stopped the spread of germs from surface to surface. But germs could still spread through the air. The answer was simple – surgeons and other surgical staff needed to wear masks that sieve germs from their breath and stop them from infecting patients.

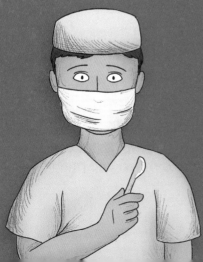

GERM ARMY

Although the vast majority of microbes are harmless, there are a great number of microbes that can make you ill. Scientists call these disease-causing microbes, or germs, 'pathogens'. The main kinds are viruses, fungi, protozoa and bacteria. Here is a round-up of some of these tiny villains.

Viruses

Viruses are much tinier than any other kind of germ. They only come to life once they have invaded and taken over a living cell, such as one of your body cells.

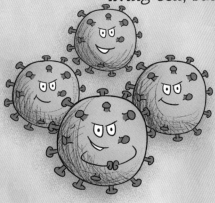

Influenza viruses give you colds and flu. Type C gives you minor colds, type B gives you winter flu, and type A bird flu.

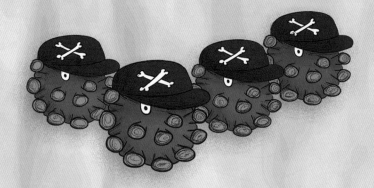

The togavirus causes rubella (German measles).

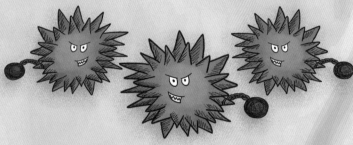

Adenoviruses give rise to sore throats, colds, bronchitis, conjunctivitis, diarrhoea and pneumonia.

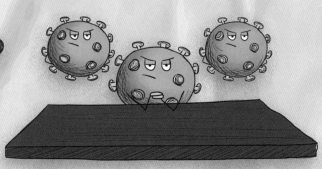

The human immuno-deficiency virus (HIV) causes AIDS.

Fungi and protozoa

A few diseases are caused by tiny organisms called fungi and protozoa.

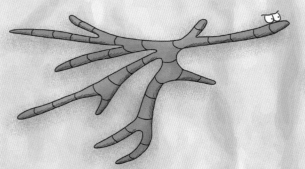

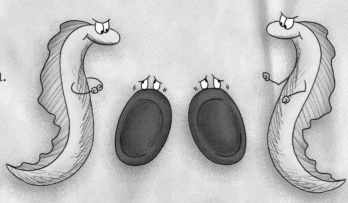

The protozoa *Trypanosoma brucei* causes sleeping sickness by attacking red blood cells.

Fungi can cause skin infections such as athlete's foot.

Bacteria

Bacteria are tiny microbes made from just one cell. Most are harmless, but a few are germs that make you ill.

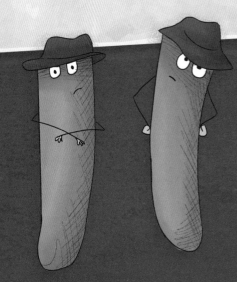

Bacilli are long, thin and rod-like, and cause tetanus (lockjaw), typhoid, tuberculosis (TB), whooping cough and diphtheria. Not welcome!

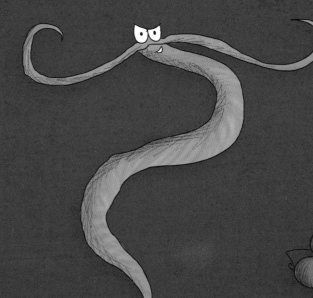

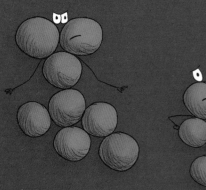

Spirilla look like tiny spiral pasta noodles and cause diarrhoea and stomach upsets.

Cocci are plump, round bacteria that cause strep throat, pneumonia, scarlet fever and meningitis.

GERMY TIMES

Some people suspected that germs caused disease long ago. Here are some of the key steps on the way to the discovery of just what germs are, and how they make you ill.

1665
Microscopic cells

English physicist Robert Hooke saw through a microscope that living things are made from tiny boxes, or 'cells'.

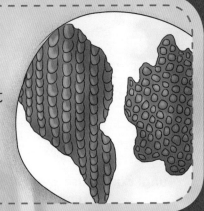

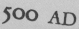

500 AD

1600

Around 1000 BC
Old herbalists

In India, the Ayurvedic system of medicine suggested that many diseases were caused by tiny microbes.

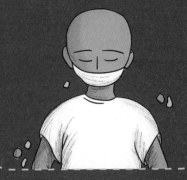

1546
The seeds of disease

Italian physician Girolamo Fracastoro suggested that diseases were spread far and wide by tiny seeds.

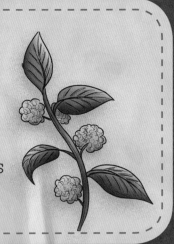

1676 Viewing bacteria

Dutch scientist Anton van Leeuwenhoek was the first person to see bacteria, through a homemade microscope.

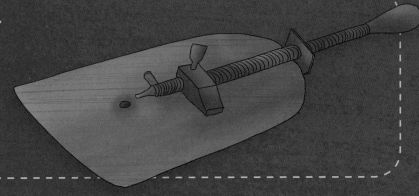

1847 Hygiene

Hungarian doctor Ignaz Semmelweis cut dangerous infections among mothers giving birth simply by getting all medical staff to wash their hands.

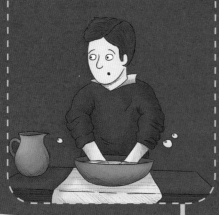

1859 Germs in the air

French microbiologist Louis Pasteur proved that there are microbes in the air that might cause disease.

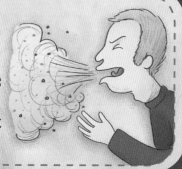

1860s Antiseptic surgery

Surgeon Joseph Lister showed how keeping everything completely clean stopped germs spreading and patients dying from infection after surgery.

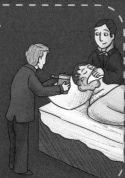

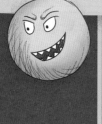

1750   1860

1876 Bacteria cause disease

German doctor Robert Koch proved that a particular bacterium caused the disease anthrax.

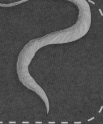

1854 Sanitation

English doctor John Snow showed that cholera was spread not by bad vapours but by sewage-contaminated water.

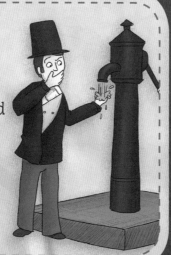

1890s Germ theory

Following on from Koch's ideas, scientists developed the germ theory: the idea that a small range of micro-organisms, known as pathogens or germs, are the cause of all infectious diseases.

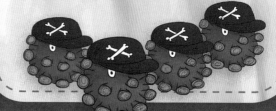

GRUESOME SYMPTOMS

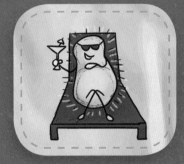

One species of bacterium is so resistant to radiation that scientists have nicknamed it 'Conan the Bacterium'.

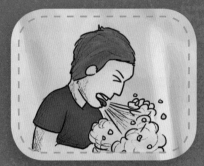

When you cough, germs can travel about three metres if you don't cover your nose or mouth with your hand or a handkerchief.

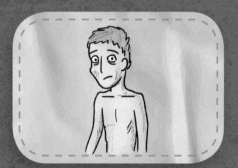

There are more bacteria in and on your body than there are people in the world. Around 1% of your body weight is bacteria.

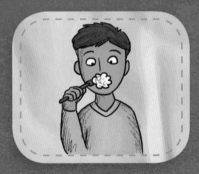

Bacteria in your nose and mouth are what give you bad breath.

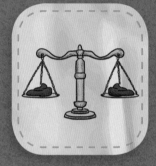

Take out the water, and around 30% of your poo is bacteria.

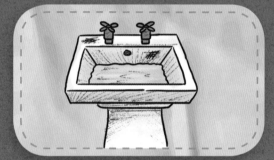

The average kitchen sink contains 100,000 times more germs than the bathroom.

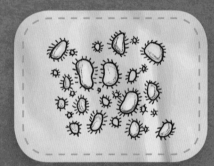

Bacteria double in number every 20 minutes. A single bacterium could divide and multiply into trillions in just one day, if all the bacteria survived.

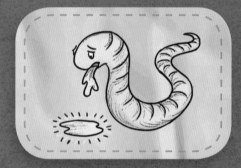

Some soldiers in the American Civil War had 'glow-in-the-dark' wounds because of a bioluminescent bacterium that was puked up by nematode worms.

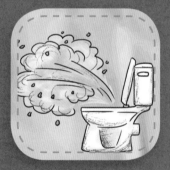

When you flush a toilet, an invisible cloud of water full of germs shoots far up into the air.

GLOSSARY

Antiseptic	A substance wiped or sprayed on surfaces to kill germs
Ayurveda	An ancient medical system developed in India that treats people with complex mixes of herbs
Bacterium	(plural: bacteria) A microbe made from just one cell
Bubonic plague	A dreadful disease caused by the bacterium *Yersinia pestis* that often leads to distinctive buboes
Epidemic	A widespread outbreak of an infectious disease
Germ	A microbe that causes disease when it enters the body
Immune system	The system by which your body protects itself against disease
Miasma	A damp, smelly mist that was believed to spread disease
Microbe	An extremely small living thing which you can only see if you use a microscope
Puerperal fever	A disease that affects mothers giving birth
Vaccination	The method of using dead or weakened germs to stimulate the body's immune system to guard against infection
Virus	A tiny germ that reproduces only inside other living cells

Index

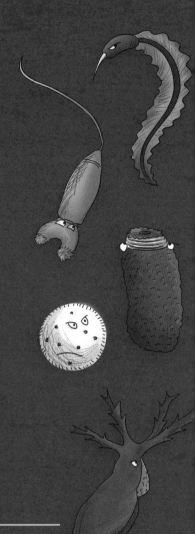

The Author

John Farndon is the author of many books on science, technology and nature, including the international best-sellers *Do Not Open* and *Do You Think You're Clever?* He has been shortlisted five times for the Royal Society's Young People's Book Prize.

The Illustrator

Venitia Dean grew up in Brighton, UK. She has loved drawing ever since she could hold a pencil. After receiving a digital drawing tablet for her 19th birthday she transferred to working digitally. She hasn't looked back since!

怪诞 医学史

致命的病菌

约翰·法恩登〔英〕 著

温妮莎·迪安〔英〕 绘

罗来鸥 译

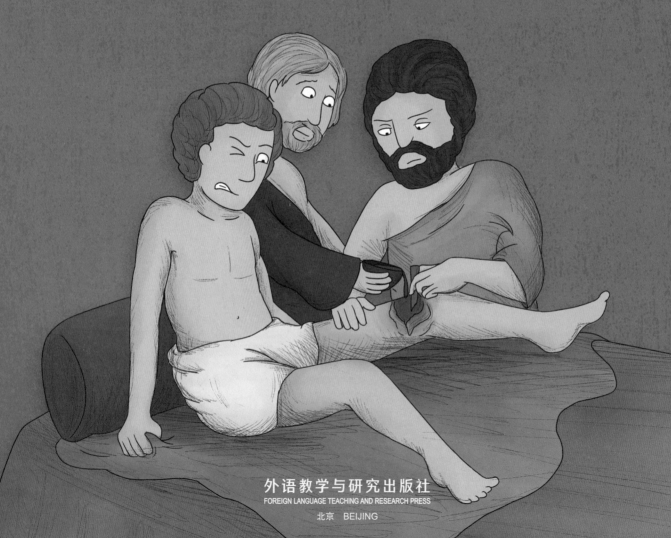

外语教学与研究出版社

FOREIGN LANGUAGE TEACHING AND RESEARCH PRESS

北京 BEIJING

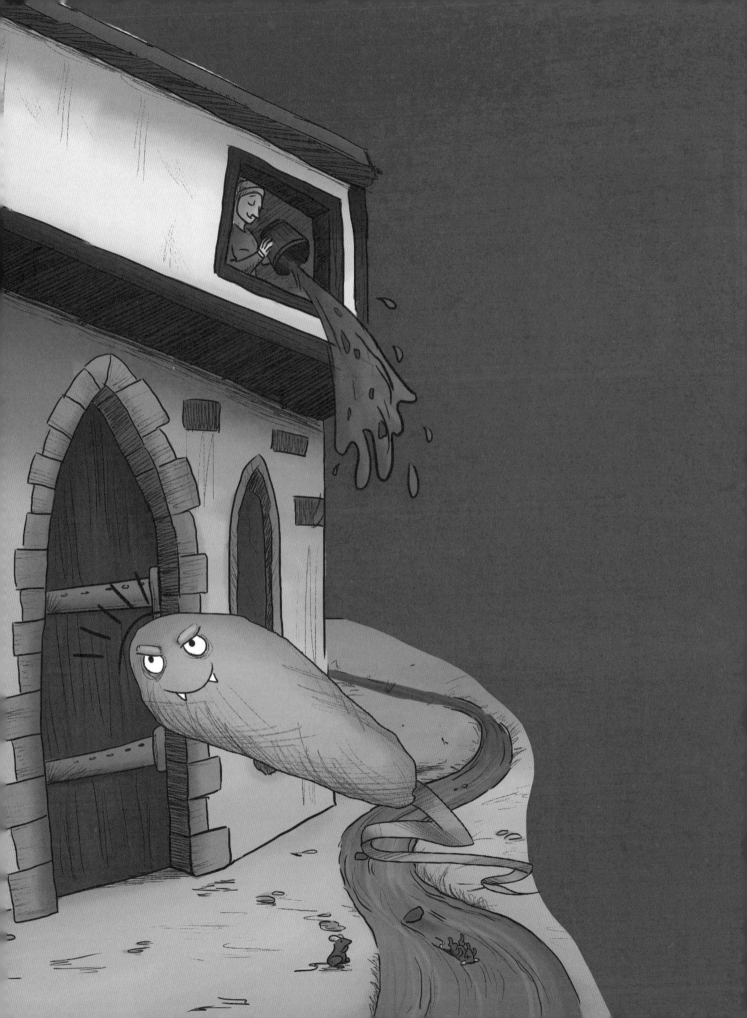

肉眼看不见的微生物在我们的身体里安营扎寨,迅速繁殖,从而引发疾病。让我们跟随这本书,了解数千年来人类如何设法追踪这些微型杀手,又如何战胜和消灭它们。

- 天花和结核病从牛身上传播
- 霍乱使人皮肤皱缩,浑身青紫
- 医院曾引发致命疾病

　　......

　　在对抗疾病的战役中,人们取得了一些伟大胜利:法国科学家路易·巴斯德揭示了病菌存在于空气中,德国医生罗伯特·科赫证明了病菌能引发疾病,英国外科医生约瑟夫·利斯特开创了在高度清洁的环境下实施手术的方法......一起来看看吧!

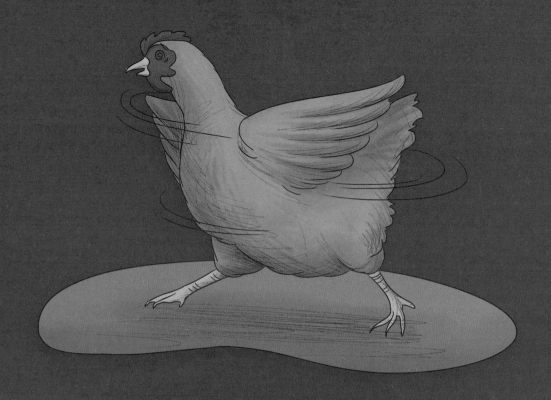

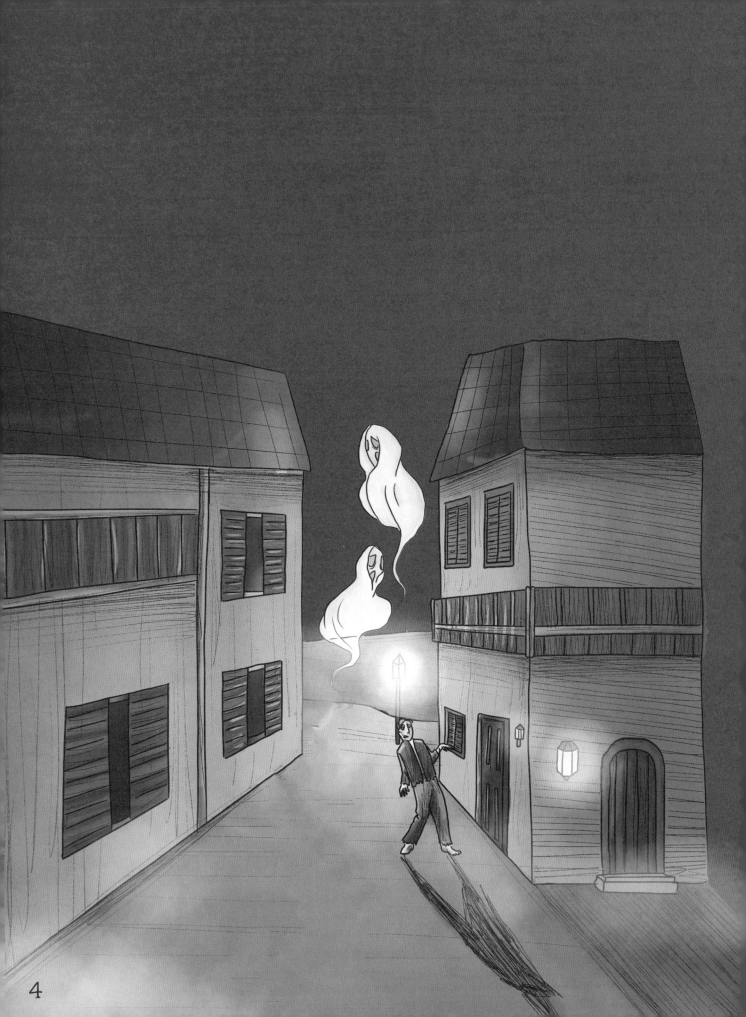

目录

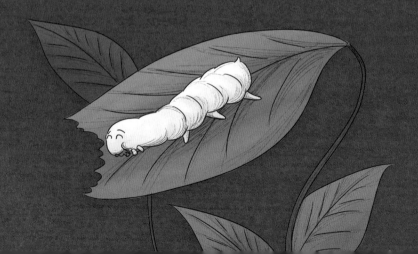

写在前面

病菌是能够使人生病的微生物，它们小到人的肉眼无法看到，因此能够在你毫无察觉的情况下悄悄潜入你的身体，让你感染上各种可怕的疾病。这本书讲的就是这些小恶魔最终是如何被人类发现和认识的。

不速之"客"

病菌并非有意让人类生病，只是我们的身体是它们非常理想的寄生家园。它们一旦进入人体，就会充分利用这个大好机会迅速繁殖，从而损害感染病菌者的身体健康。

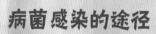

病菌感染的途径

病菌遍及世界各地的各种场所。一些病菌在空气中通过人的喷嚏、咳嗽或呼吸进入人体。如果你用手触碰了被病菌污染的东西，接着又摸鼻子、吸气，那么你可能就会感染病菌。还有一些病菌附着在不干净或者腐败变质的食物上，如果你吃了这类东西，病菌就会随之溜进你的肚子。

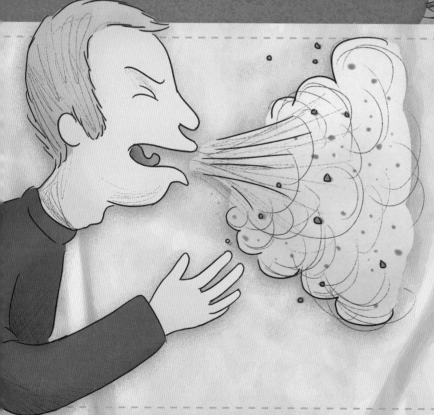

人体中的卫士

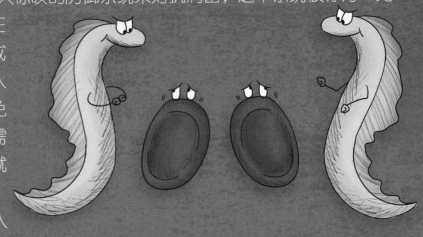

万分幸运的是，人体拥有令人惊叹的防御系统来对抗病菌，这个系统被称为"免疫系统"。它实际上是一支由在血液中游弋的众多微小细胞组成的复杂军团，这个军团会向侵入人体的病菌发起进攻。但是，免疫系统在人体遭受病菌侵袭后需要一段时间才能发挥作用，这就是为什么我们会生病。生病后，如果运气好，免疫系统打败了入侵的敌人，我们就会恢复健康。

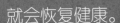

医生的治病"法宝"

医生有两种方式帮助你的身体战胜病菌。一种方式是疫苗接种，通过注射疫苗刺激人体免疫系统进入"备战"状态，抵御特定种类的病菌；另一种方式是使用抗生素，这种化学物质通常被制成口服药片。对病菌来说，抗生素就是消灭它们的"毒药"。

保持清洁的重要性

另外还有一种办法可以减少病菌侵害，这个办法就是保持环境清洁卫生。因为许多病菌都是在肮脏污秽的环境中传播，保持干净卫生就可以降低感染病菌的概率。所以说，经常洗手很有好处。

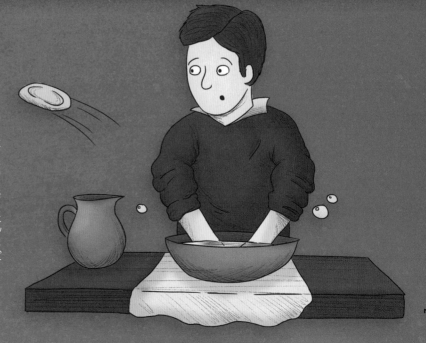

定居与病菌传播

在人类历史的早期阶段，我们的祖先居无定所，为了狩猎和采集食物不断迁徙，因此可能很少有传染病流行。那个时候，人们居住地分散，不利于病菌的传播；人们也不会长期在水源地附近居留，所以不会污染水源。

疾病流行的农场

距今大约10,000年的时候，人类文明发展到了农耕阶段，人类摆脱了饥饿的威胁，农作物又保证了早期城镇的食物供应。但是，我们现在已经知道，农耕环境下人和家畜混居，相互感染病菌，水源也遭到了污染，从而使病菌大量滋生。

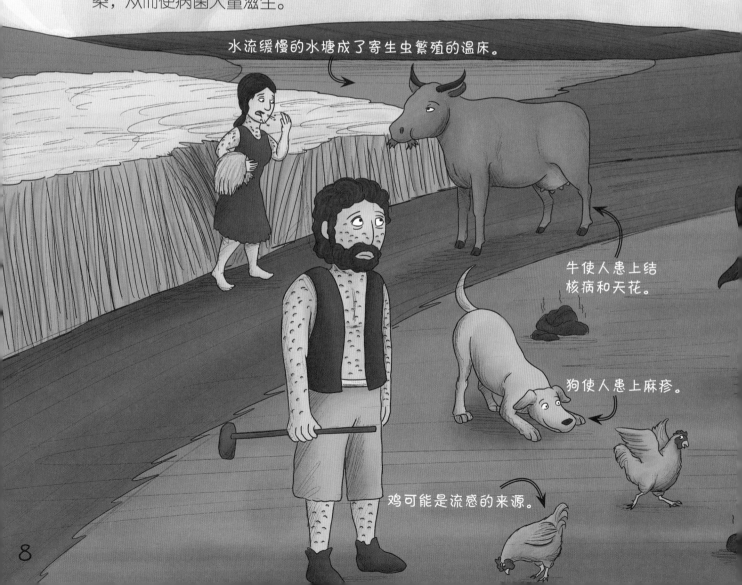

水流缓慢的水塘成了寄生虫繁殖的温床。

牛使人患上结核病和天花。

狗使人患上麻疹。

鸡可能是流感的来源。

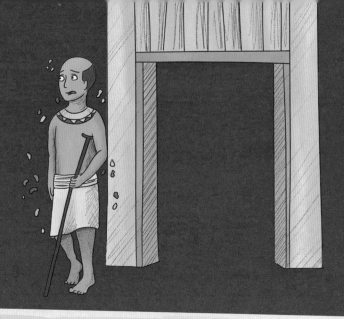

最早的脊髓灰质炎患者

3,000多年前的一块埃及石碑上有一幅画，画中的男人拄着一根手杖。他的一条腿看起来萎缩了，可能是脊髓灰质炎（也就是小儿麻痹症）导致的。如果确实如此，他就是人类已知最早患上这种可怕病症的人。引发这种病的病毒可能是在被家畜粪便污染的水源里滋生的。

随着农耕活动越来越密集，水源被粪肥污染，因此助长了脊髓灰质炎、霍乱、伤寒、肝炎等传染病的传播。水流缓慢的灌溉渠也成了寄生虫滋生的温床。这些寄生虫中，有些会使人患上血吸虫病和疟疾。

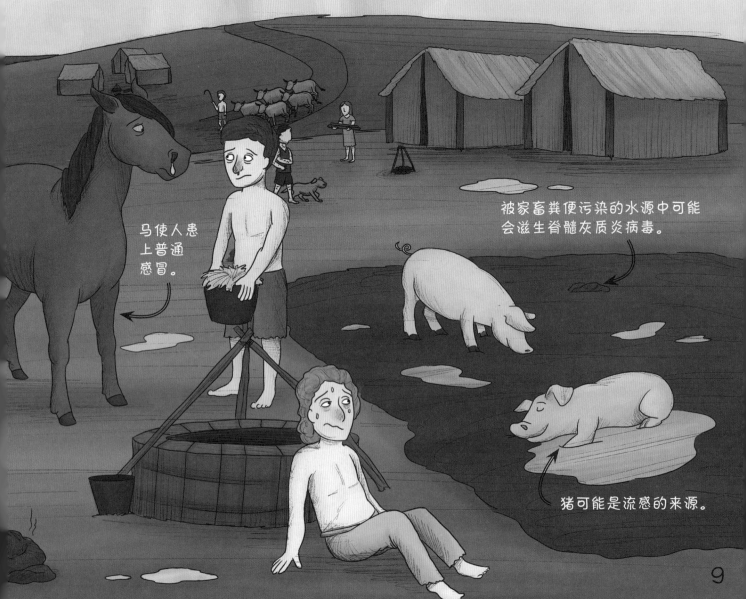

马使人患上普通感冒。

被家畜粪便污染的水源中可能会滋生脊髓灰质炎病毒。

猪可能是流感的来源。

"背黑锅"的污浊空气

过去很少有人知道疾病是通过看不见的微小病菌传播的，大多数人认为气味难闻的污浊空气是致病元凶，特别是沟渠和沼泽附近那种湿漉漉、雾蒙蒙的空气。人们把这种污浊难闻的雾气称为"瘴气"。

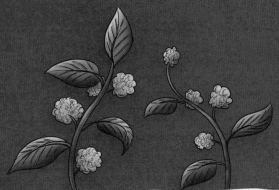

吃叶子解毒

和世界上其他地区一样，古印度大部分人也认为疾病是有毒空气造成的。他们会咀嚼用黑儿茶叶子制成的糊糊来解毒。

裹挟"毒气"的晨风

古罗马作家维特鲁威坚信，在沼泽附近兴建城市是非常不明智的。因为他认为，清晨的微风会把湿地中的瘴气和沼泽生物呼出的有毒气体吹到城市上空，致使人们生病。

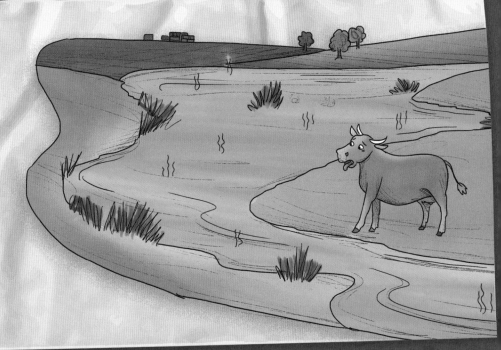

凶多吉少南方行

在古代中国，政府官员如果被朝廷流放至南方山区，他们一般都会觉得自己倒了大霉。因为南方山区通常潮湿多雾，人们深信那里的有毒空气会让人染病丧命。

新奥尔良的"邪恶"雾气

新奥尔良市曾经经常有疾病暴发。人们坚信这是附近沼泽上空充斥着邪恶幽灵的浊气带来的灾难。因此，他们燃烧大堆的小白菊，并向沼泽发射炮弹，希望能借此防止邪恶雾气的侵袭。

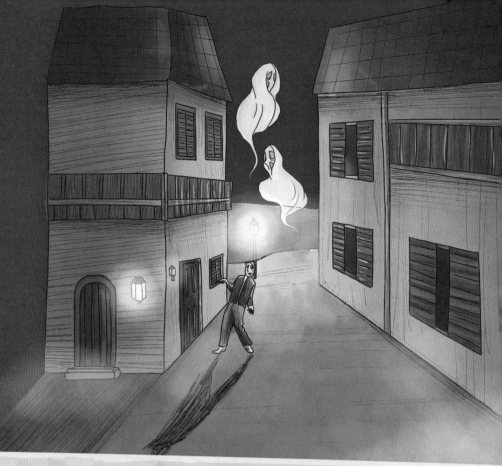

饮用被污染的河水可能会送命。

恶臭熏天的泰晤士河

在伦敦，当地的人们曾经把大量污水排进泰晤士河。这导致了在1858年的盛夏，泰晤士河散发出极其难闻的恶臭，甚至到了令人恶心呕吐的程度，史称"大恶臭"。这一局面导致一些居民逃离伦敦城，因为他们坚信，污水散发出的难闻臭气会让人染上致命疾病。为了解决这个问题，伦敦建立了全世界第一个现代污水处理系统。

东方人对病菌的认识

你或许会认为，过去的人们对病菌一无所知，因为它们太小，无法被肉眼看到。但早在几千年前的印度，耆那教信徒就已经被灌输了一种观念：人们被一种四面八方无处不在的微小生命形态包围着，这种生命形态被称为"尼俱陀"。

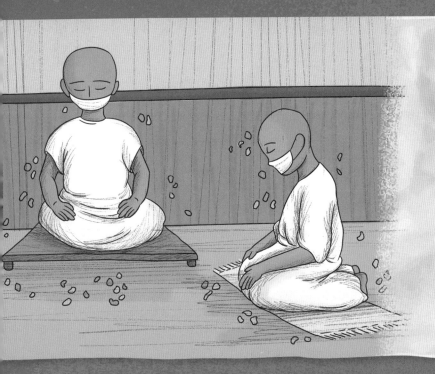

避免杀生的口罩

如今，为了避免吸入病菌，人们经常会戴上医用口罩。几千年前的耆那教信徒也会戴口罩，但他们这样做不是为了避免生病，而是他们信奉绝不杀生的原则，不想在不经意间吞入无处不在的"尼俱陀"而让这些微小生物送命。

古老的传统医学

阿育吠陀医学体系历史悠久，它诞生于3,000多年前的印度，使用配方复杂的草药来医治病人。科学家们无法确定这一医学体系的科学性，但直到现在仍有不少人使用阿育吠陀疗法治病。研习阿育吠陀医学的医生们那时就认为，微生物会引发麻风病、脑膜炎等疾病。

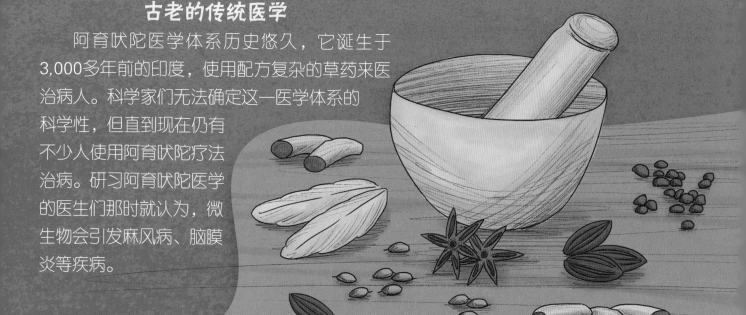

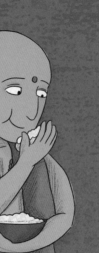

预防胜于治疗

大约2,000年前由阇罗迦编纂的《阇罗迦本集》是最重要的阿育吠陀医学古代著作之一。该著作中提到预防胜于治疗，因此，为了保持身体健康，在不同的地域和一年中的不同时节要吃不同的食物。

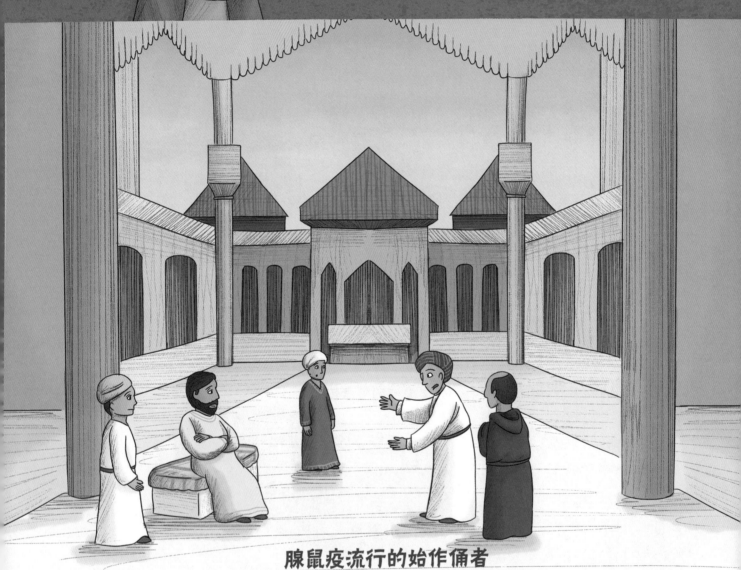

腺鼠疫流行的始作俑者

1350年前后，腺鼠疫疫情扩散至西班牙的格拉纳达，之后疫情又在部分伊斯兰国家出现。医师伊本·哈提马认为，是一种"微小体"造成了腺鼠疫的流行。这种"微小体"听起来很像我们现在所说的病菌。另一位医师哈提卜（图中戴橙色头巾的人，图中宫殿是格拉纳达的艾勒汉卜拉宫，听他说话的人是一位国家高官），则解释了这种"微小体"如何通过人与人之间的接触来传播腺鼠疫。

隐形生物显形记

大概在1590年，荷兰眼镜制作师扎哈里亚斯·扬森把几片透镜放到一起，发明了显微镜。当人们通过这种显微镜观察时，被眼前的一切惊呆了：他们看到了一个不为人知的全新微生物世界，这些微生物很小，无法直接用肉眼看到。

细胞的发现

1665年，英格兰物理学家罗伯特·胡克（1635—1703）发表了《显微图谱》，这本书汇集了他所绘制的通过显微镜观察到的种种奇妙个体，这些个体都是人们以前从来没有见过的。从一些软木薄片上，胡克还观察到像蜂巢一般纵横交错排列的一个个小盒子，他称这些盒子为"细胞"。我们现在已经知道，所有的生物都是由一个个微小的细胞构成的。

万千"鬼怪"现原形

荷兰科学家安东·范·列文虎克（1632—1723）制成了只有一个透镜镜片的显微镜。这个显微镜构造简单，但效果极佳，用它能够看到放大了200倍的。通过显微镜的观察，列文虎克发现清水其实并不"清"，而是充满了微生物。实际上，这些微生物几乎是无处不在的。

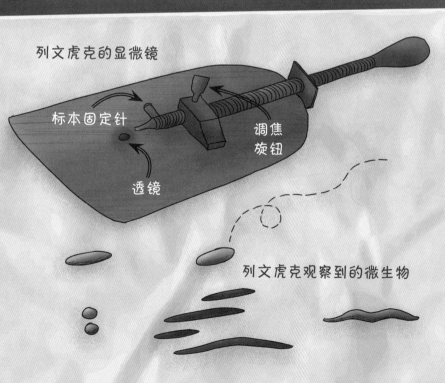

列文虎克的显微镜

标本固定针

调焦旋钮

透镜

列文虎克观察到的微生物

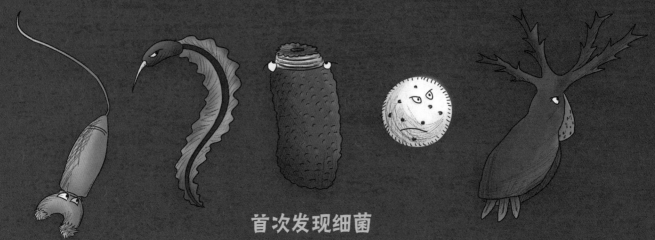

首次发现细菌

列文虎克观察到了形态各异的微生物（如上图）后感到非常吃惊，这些微生物中有很多外表很可怕。列文虎克是最早观察到细菌的人。他在用显微镜观察从人的牙齿上取下的牙菌斑时，看到了蠕动的细菌。

科恩的发现：细菌的四种主要形态

虽然列文虎克的发现堪称伟大，但其后的200年间并没有人对细菌给予密切关注。直到19世纪70年代，德国生物学家费迪南德·科恩才开始对细菌进行深入研究。科恩发现，虽然细菌的种类很多，但根据它们的形状，他可以把这些细菌划分为四大类，即球状细菌、杆状细菌、丝状细菌和螺旋状细菌。

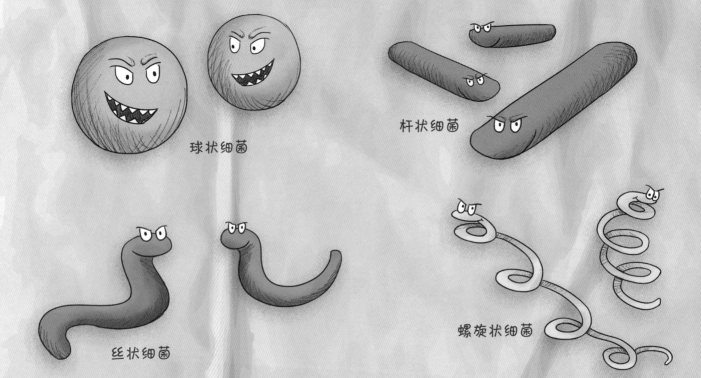

球状细菌

杆状细菌

丝状细菌

螺旋状细菌

洗手等于救命

过去的医院是病人九死一生的地方。那时几乎没有人知道病菌会使人生病，医生和护士在接触了一个又一个病人的同时也造成了疾病的传播，后果非常严重。

"不要把我送进医院!"

以前，在家分娩对于年轻妈妈们来说绝非易事。但如果去医院，她们面临的则很可能是生命危险。医生们的双手会沾带上致命病菌——产褥热病菌，从而使一个又一个年轻妈妈被传染。所以，去医院分娩对当时的产妇来说可能等于被宣判了死刑。

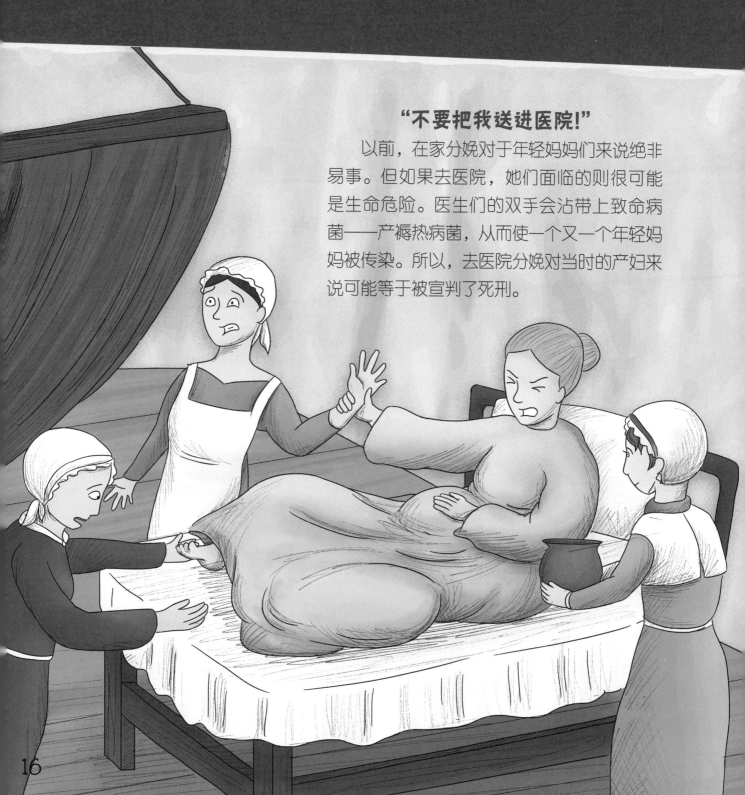

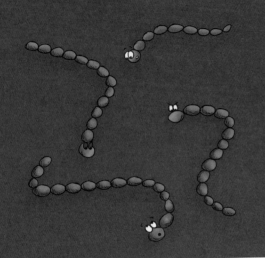

揪出真凶

当然，真正应该被怪罪的不是医生。他们没有清洗的手沾染了病菌，而这些病菌才是真正的元凶。如今我们已经知道，导致产妇患上产褥热的病菌是一种名为"化脓性链球菌"的细菌。幸运的是，如果医院卫生条件良好，这种病菌就几乎不会有逞凶的机会。

救人还是害人？

在19世纪的维也纳总医院，医生常常会在处理完太平间的病人尸体后，转身就进入产科第一产房去为产妇检查身体，造成了产妇大量死亡。1847年，当年轻的匈牙利医生伊格纳茨·塞麦尔维斯（1818—1865）来到医院时，产房里的高死亡率让他震惊，后来他意识到这是医生的问题。

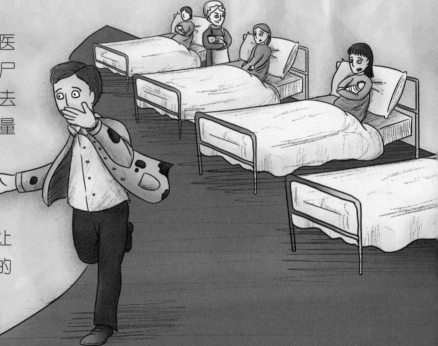

"我的手洗干净了！"

塞麦尔维斯要求所有的医护人员定期用氯化钙溶液洗手。这一举措实施后，产科第一产房的死亡率立刻有所下降。但医生们无法相信是他们导致了产妇的死亡，于是他们解雇了塞麦尔维斯，不再要求医护人员洗手，仍然一切照旧。又过了一段时间，人们才真正认识到保持清洁卫生对于遏制病菌传播的重要性。

"藏污纳垢"的下水道

19世纪的时候，伦敦和其他欧洲城市迅速发展，致命传染病霍乱
所导致的死亡人数也随之迅速增加，穷人感染霍乱的情况尤为严重。

折磨人的霍乱

霍乱是一种可怕的疾病，可能起源于印度恒河沿岸地区。感染了霍乱的人会严重腹泻，造成身体脱水。他们会变得眼神空洞无光，皮肤皱缩，浑身青紫。

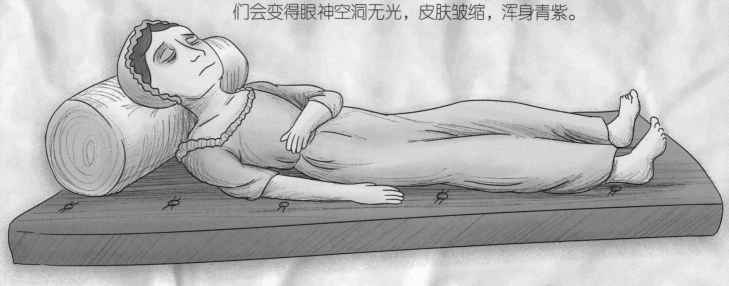

哪里来的臭气？

过去的专家们坚信是瘴气造成了霍乱的蔓延。因此，那些上流社会的人想当然地认为，这是身上散发着难闻气味的穷人们的过错。当时的一幅漫画讽刺了那些试图嗅探出恶臭来源的主管卫生的官老爷们。

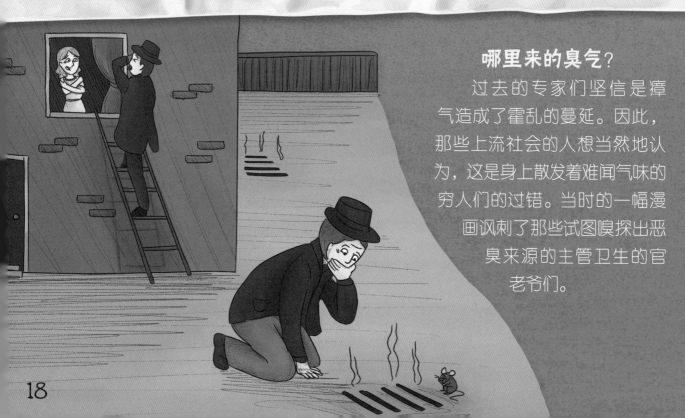

索霍区的水泵

英格兰医生约翰·斯诺并不认同"瘴气致病"理论。1854年,当霍乱在伦敦索霍区肆虐时,他发现所有感染者都喝了布罗德维克街同一个水泵的水,而这个水泵的供水水源已经被人的粪便污染。然而,多年以后人们才认识到霍乱是由脏水中的病菌引发的。

交通发展加剧疫情传播

1869年,埃及苏伊士运河通航。它大大缩短了印度到欧洲的航程,同时也使霍乱的传播变得更加容易。那时的伦敦已经建立了完善的污水处理系统,因而避免了霍乱在此酿成严重的后果,但是欧洲其他城市却饱受霍乱肆虐之苦。

可怕的霍乱弧菌

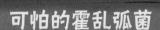

1854年,也就是伦敦索霍区出现霍乱疫情的同年,霍乱也席卷了意大利佛罗伦萨。在这里,微生物学家菲利波·帕奇尼通过显微镜发现了致病元凶——霍乱弧菌。但是他的发现并没有受到人们的重视,大家仍然认为瘴气是真凶。1883年,德国医生罗伯特·科赫(1843—1910)也认定霍乱弧菌是人感染霍乱的罪魁祸首。由于科赫声名远播,这次人们都相信了他关于霍乱弧菌的说法。

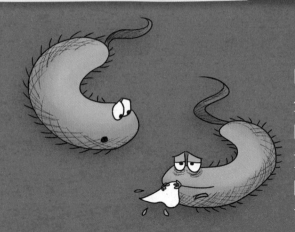

巴斯德的实验与免疫研究

19世纪40年代和50年代，塞麦尔维斯和斯诺两位医生向人们证明，保持双手清洁和完善排水设施可以阻止疾病传播。如此看来，认为污浊空气造成传染病流行的说法是站不住脚的。到19世纪60年代，法国微生物学家路易·巴斯德（1822—1895）开始用他的研究论证，造成疾病流行的真凶是微生物。

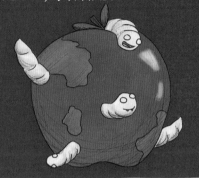

自然发生说

过去，当人们看到蛆虫从烂苹果或腐肉里蠕动着爬出来时，不会想到它们是从卵孵化而来的，而是觉得这些蛆虫就是在食物腐烂时凭空冒出来的。这种认为生命毫无来源、凭空出现的观点被称为"自然发生说"。

空气中的微生物

1859年，巴斯德用一个简单的实验证明，食物腐烂时，微生物不是通过自然发生的方法像变戏法似的变出来的，而是来自于空气中的灰尘。

1. 巴斯德将肉汤盛在一个瓶颈细长且弯曲的鹅颈瓶里，加热至沸腾，以杀死里面的微生物。

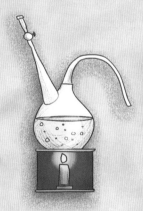

2. 鹅颈瓶的瓶颈阻止灰尘落入，因此汤水保持清澈。

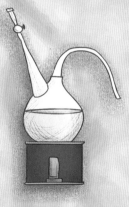

3. 巴斯德将瓶颈打断，灰尘落入，肉汤很快就变浑浊，这说明微生物开始繁殖。

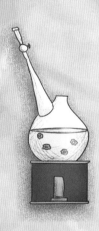

杀死蚕宝宝的微生物

1867年，巴斯德证明了微生物可以引发疾病。他此前一直在研究一种导致蚕宝宝死亡的病症。当巴斯德通过显微镜观察那些染病的蚕宝宝时，他发现它们感染上的不止是一种微生物，而是两种。

20

鸡霍乱菌实验

1879年，巴斯德通过在鸡身上做实验，发现了保护人们不被病菌感染的方法。他用培养皿培养鸡霍乱菌，然后通过阻断养分供应的方式使病菌的活性减弱，降低其毒性。之后他将这些毒性减弱的病菌注入实验用鸡的体内，鸡就对霍乱产生了免疫。如今，接种毒性减弱的病菌制成的疫苗是人类预防疾病的主要方式之一。

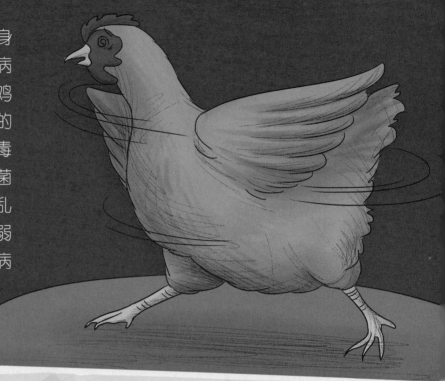

给羊接种

1881年，巴斯德还找到了一种方法，来减弱使羊感染炭疽的病菌的毒性。巴斯德使用这些病菌毒性减弱了的疫苗给羊接种，羊就对炭疽产生了免疫。

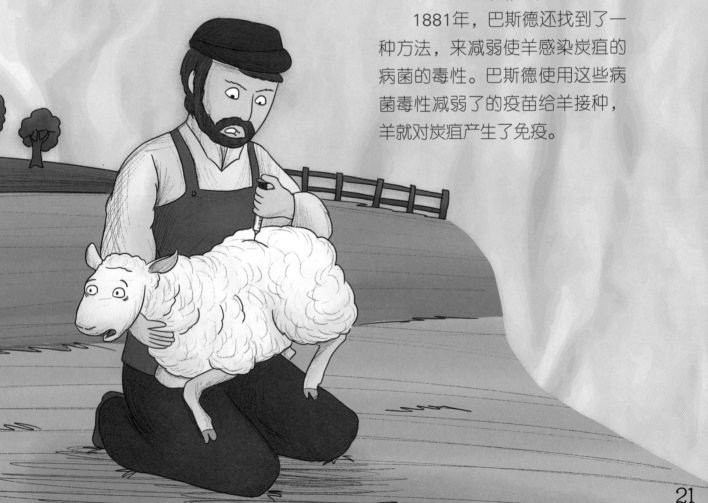

锁定致病真凶

路易·巴斯德证明了空气中有微生物，并且这些微生物可以引发疾病。后来，罗伯特·科赫又向人们揭示，这支可恶的微生物大军规模庞大——大多数疾病的致病元凶正是这些可恶的微生物。

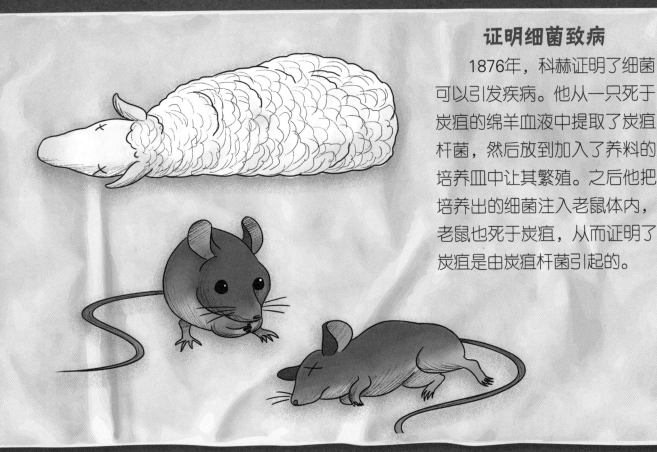

证明细菌致病

1876年，科赫证明了细菌可以引发疾病。他从一只死于炭疽的绵羊血液中提取了炭疽杆菌，然后放到加入了养料的培养皿中让其繁殖。之后他把培养出的细菌注入老鼠体内，老鼠也死于炭疽，从而证明了炭疽是由炭疽杆菌引起的。

夺命杀手——炭疽杆菌

炭疽杆菌是一种杆状微生物，它极其微小，需要在显微镜下才能看到。虽然它很小，却能杀死一只羊，甚至会使人送命。这种细菌可以在宿主体内非常快速地繁殖并释放毒素，从而对宿主造成危害。

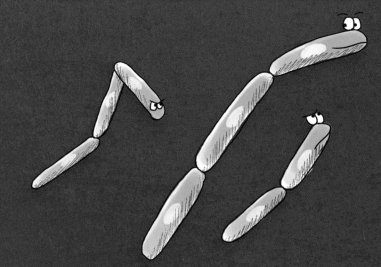

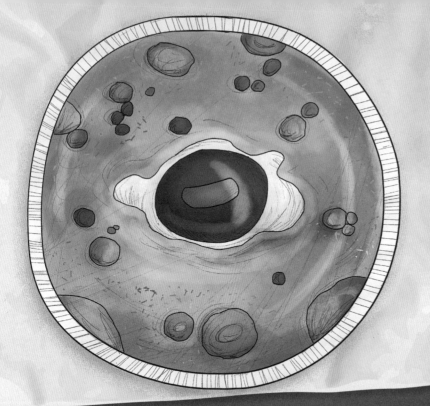

病菌培养

科赫的病菌研究需要在实验室里用培养皿培养病菌，像这样被培养出来的病菌被称为"培养物"，它们需要养料。起初，科赫使用公牛眼部分泌的液体作为病菌培养物的养料。后来他又研制出了一种汤汁，这种汤汁的成分为琼脂（一种取自海藻的胶质物）和明胶（一种取自动物骨头的胶质物）。

科赫法则的四步验证

科赫通过研究设计了四个验证步骤，用来验证某一种疾病对应的病菌。

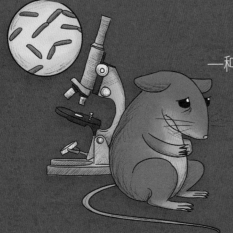

1. 关联验证：该病菌总是在患某一病症的动物身上发现。

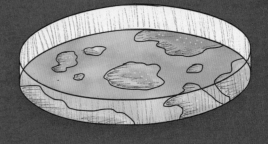

2. 分离验证：该病菌可从患病动物体内提取，并作为纯培养物培养。

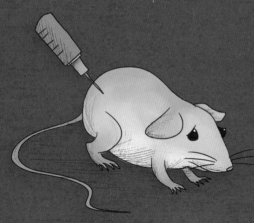

3. 接种验证：从患病动物体内提取的该病菌能使健康动物患同种病症。

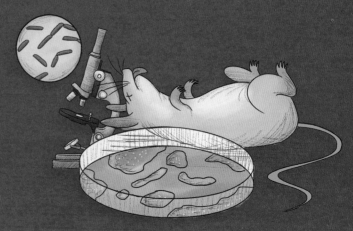

4. 再分离验证：在因接种而新染病的动物体内也能提取到这种病菌。

病菌感染与手术消毒

如果病菌能使人染病，那如何能避免病菌感染呢？答案之一就是保持清洁卫生。塞麦尔维斯向人们证明了产妇分娩时卫生的重要性。英国外科医生约瑟夫·利斯特（1827—1912）也证明了干净卫生的手术环境对手术至关重要。

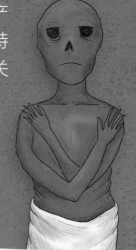

木乃伊长久保存的奥秘

尸体会因为受到微生物的侵袭而腐烂，不过古埃及人知道如何把尸体制成木乃伊来防腐。他们将尸体浸入防腐液中，利用这些防腐液的毒性杀死微生物。

流脓不是好兆头

13世纪，来自卢卡的外科医生休意识到了伤口感染的危险性，于是他用酒来清洗伤口。他发现伤口流脓不是好现象，因为这说明伤口出现了感染。而那时候，大多数医生错误地认为流脓是伤情好转的征兆。

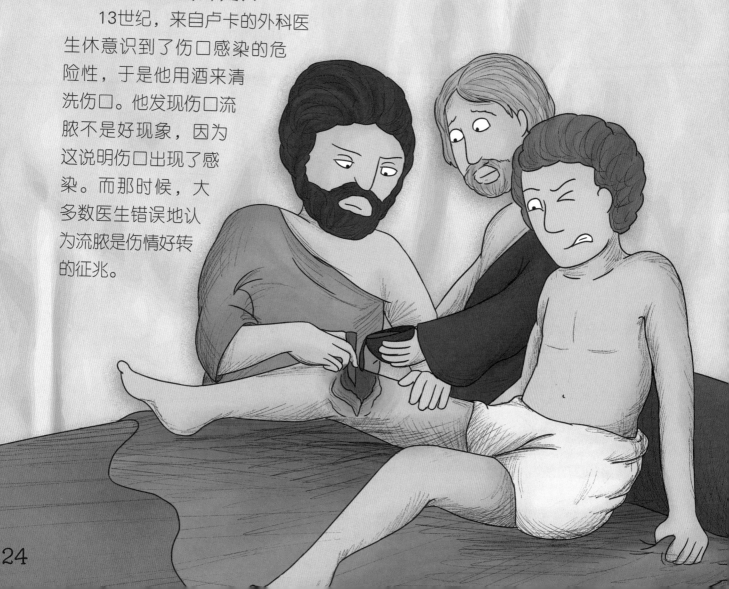

污秽不堪的城市

19世纪，快速发展中的城市肮脏不堪，因为这时的城市垃圾收集处理系统尚不完备，供水不足，排水设施也不完善。在这样的条件下，病菌很容易传播。聚集着大量污秽物的医院也是那些不爱干净的病菌最爱光顾的地方之一！

手术消毒操作

19世纪60年代之前，大量接受手术的病人死于术后感染。后来，约瑟夫·利斯特提出了外科手术需要使用消毒剂进行消毒操作的主张。他在手术前会确保使用可杀菌的化学制品——比如石炭酸皂——对手术人员的双手、手术器具和操作台表面彻底消毒。利斯特的这一消毒理念非常有效，而彻底消毒如今也已经成为全世界通用的手术操作规范。

口罩防护

利斯特的消毒措施阻止了病菌在物体表面间的传播，但是病菌还可以通过空气传播。阻止病菌在空气中传播的办法也很简单——执行手术的外科医生和其他手术人员需要佩戴口罩，来过滤他们呼出的病菌，阻止病菌通过医护人员的呼吸感染病人。

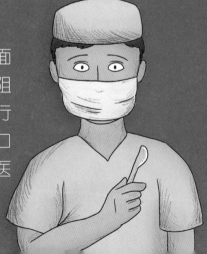

病菌的主要类型

虽然绝大多数的微生物都是无害的，但致病微生物的数量也很庞大。科学家们把这些致病微生物——或者说病菌——命名为"病原体"，它们主要包括病毒、真菌、原生动物和细菌。下面我们就来认识一下这些微型杀手中的部分成员。

病毒

病毒比其他任何一种病菌都要微小。它们只有在入侵并占据活细胞——比如人体中的细胞——之后才具备活性。

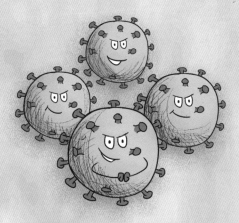

流感病毒会使人患感冒和流感。其中，丙型流感病毒会引发轻微感冒；乙型流感病毒会引发冬季流感；甲型流感病毒会引发禽流感。

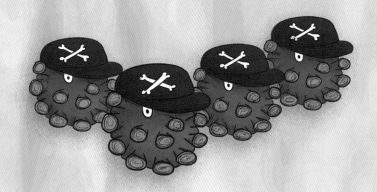

披膜病毒会引发风疹（又名德国麻疹）。

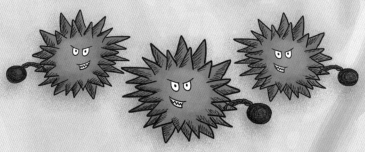

腺病毒会引发咽喉疼痛、感冒、支气管炎、结膜炎、腹泻和肺炎。

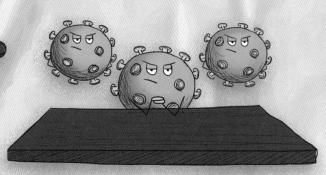

人类免疫缺陷病毒会引发艾滋病。

真菌和原生动物

有些疾病是真菌和原生动物这两种微生物引发的。

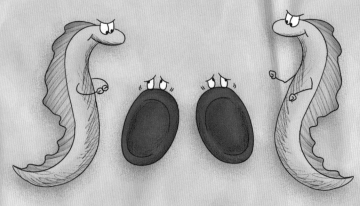

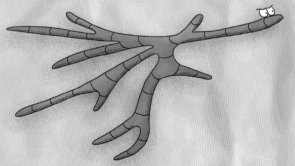

原生动物布氏锥虫会通过攻击血液中的红细胞来引发昏睡病。

真菌会引发足癣等皮肤病。

细菌

细菌是单细胞微生物，大多数无害，但有一小部分属于病菌，会使人生病。

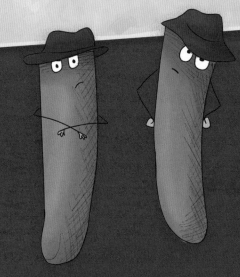

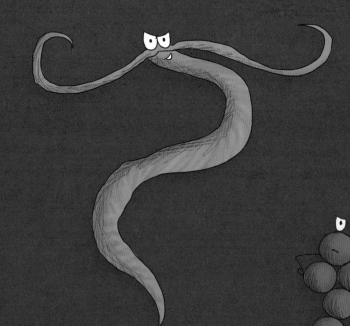

杆菌是细长的杆形细菌，会引发破伤风（又名牙关紧闭症）、伤寒、结核病、百日咳和白喉。它们是不受欢迎的家伙。

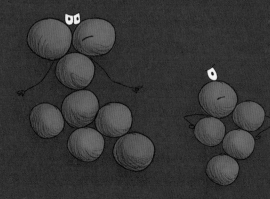

螺菌看起来像螺旋形的小号意大利面，会导致腹泻和肠胃不适。

球菌是一种形状圆鼓鼓的细菌，会引发链球菌性咽喉炎、肺炎、猩红热和脑膜炎。

27

回看人类认识病菌的历程

很早以前就有人怀疑病菌能引发疾病。以下记录的，是人们在逐渐认识病菌是什么以及病菌如何致病的历程中的一些里程碑事件。

1665年
显微镜下观察到细胞
英格兰物理学家罗伯特·胡克通过显微镜观察到生物是由一个个小盒子——细胞——构成的。

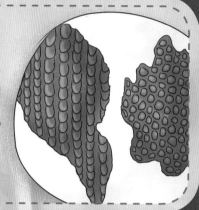

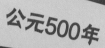
公元500年

1600年

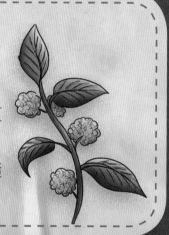

约公元前1000年
草药医生的推断
在印度，研习阿育吠陀医学的医生提出，很多疾病的致病元凶是微生物。

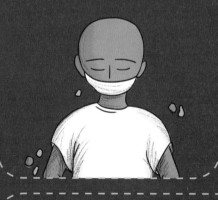

1546年
提出"致病种子"的想法
意大利医师吉罗拉莫·弗拉卡斯托罗提出，是微小的"致病种子"造成了传染病的广泛传播。

1676年
细菌现形
荷兰科学家安东·范·列文虎克通过自制的显微镜观察到了细菌，成为第一个观察到细菌的人。

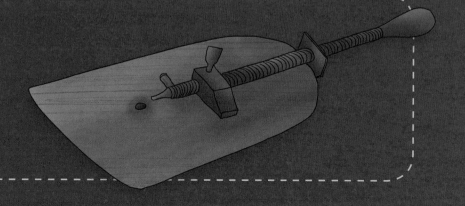

1847年
个人卫生引起重视
匈牙利医生伊格纳茨·塞麦尔维斯仅仅通过让医护人员洗手，就大幅降低了产妇出现致命感染的概率。

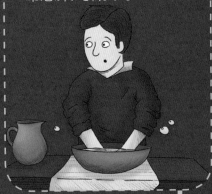

1859年
发现空气中存在病菌
法国微生物学家路易·巴斯德证明了空气中含有可能引发疾病的微生物。

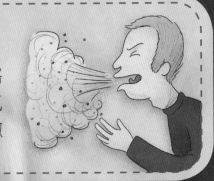

19世纪60年代
手术消毒开始应用
外科医生约瑟夫·利斯特用实践展示了将手术室中的一切物品彻底消毒可以阻止病菌传播，防止病人死于术后感染。

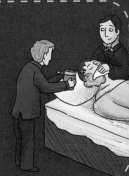

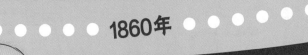

1750年   1860年

1876年
细菌致病被证实
德国医生罗伯特·科赫证明了炭疽的致病元凶是一种特定的细菌——炭疽杆菌。

1854年
公共卫生引发关注
英格兰医生约翰·斯诺向世人揭示，霍乱的传播途径是受污染的水，而非浊气。

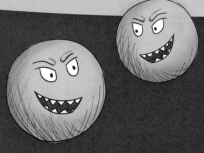

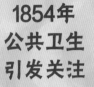

19世纪90年代
病菌理论建立
在科赫所提出观点的基础上，科学家们建立了一套病菌理论：一小部分被称为病原体或病菌的微生物是引发所有传染性疾病的罪魁祸首。

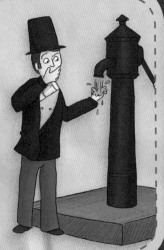

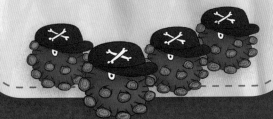

微生物趣味小百科

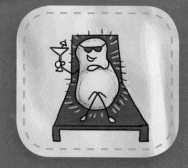

有一种细菌对辐射有极强的耐受力，科学家戏称其为"细菌柯南"（美国电影《野蛮人柯南》中的柯南本领高超、英勇无敌，译注）。

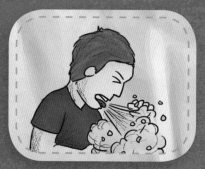

咳嗽时，如果不用手或手帕遮挡口鼻部位，咳出的病菌可以传播到大约三米远的地方。

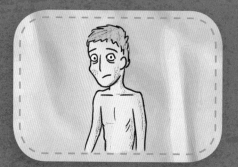

人体内和体表的细菌数量超过全世界所有人口的数量。人体重量的约1%是细菌的重量。

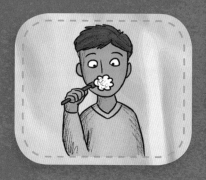

口臭是由鼻子和嘴巴里的细菌导致的。

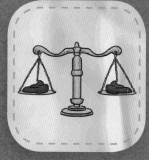

除去水分，细菌约占人粪便的30%。

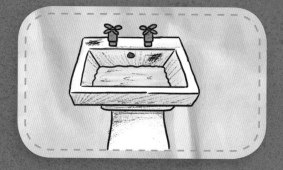

一般来说，厨房水槽中的病菌数量比卫生间的多十万倍。

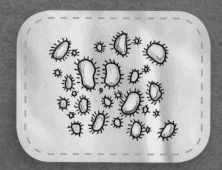

细菌的数量每20分钟就可以增加一倍。假使繁殖的每一代细菌都能存活，那么单个细菌在一天内可以分裂繁殖出数万亿个新细菌。

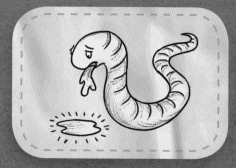

美国南北战争时期，一些受伤军人的伤口会在黑暗中"发光"，这是由于伤口被线虫吐出的发光菌所感染。

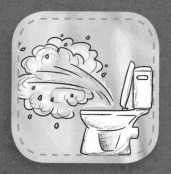

冲马桶时，会高高溅起肉眼看不到的、充斥着病菌的水雾。

术语表

阿育吠陀医学体系	源于印度的一种古代医学体系，使用配方复杂的草药来医治病人
病毒	只能靠寄生在其他生物的活细胞内繁殖的微小病菌
病菌	进入体内后能引发疾病的微生物
产褥热	产妇在产褥期患的一种疾病
流行病	暴发后广泛蔓延的传染性疾病
免疫系统	人体自身对抗疾病的系统
微生物	一种极小的、需要用显微镜观察的生物
细菌	一种单细胞微生物
腺鼠疫	由鼠疫杆菌引发的可怕疾病，其特征是感染者常常会出现腹股沟淋巴结炎
消毒剂	涂抹或喷洒到物体表面用于杀死病菌的物质
疫苗接种	接种失去活性或活性减弱的病菌以刺激免疫系统产生应答，从而预防感染的防疫方法
瘴气	一种具有难闻气味的潮湿雾气，旧时被认为能传播疾病

索引

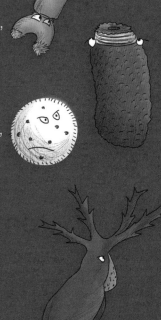

作者简介

约翰·法恩登是位多产的科普图书作家，作品涉及科学、技术和自然领域，包括全球畅销书《放我出去》和《你觉得自己聪明吗？》，并曾五次获得英国皇家学会青少年科学图书奖的提名。

绘者简介

温妮莎·迪安成长于英国布赖顿，从小时候能握住铅笔起就十分热爱绘画。她在19岁生日时收到了一个电子绘画板，便开始尝试电子绘画，从此在这条路上探索不止。

The Grisly History of Medicine
Plague!

Written by John Farndon
Illustrated by Venitia Dean

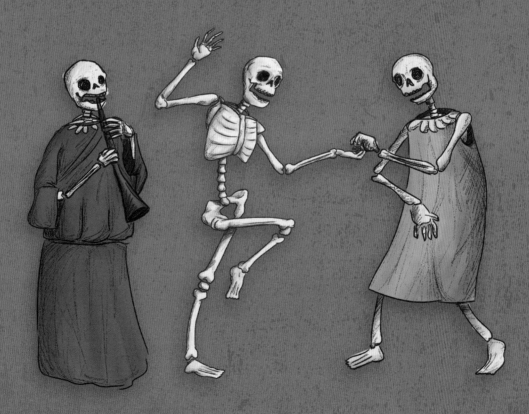

外语教学与研究出版社
FOREIGN LANGUAGE TEACHING AND RESEARCH PRESS
北京　BEIJING

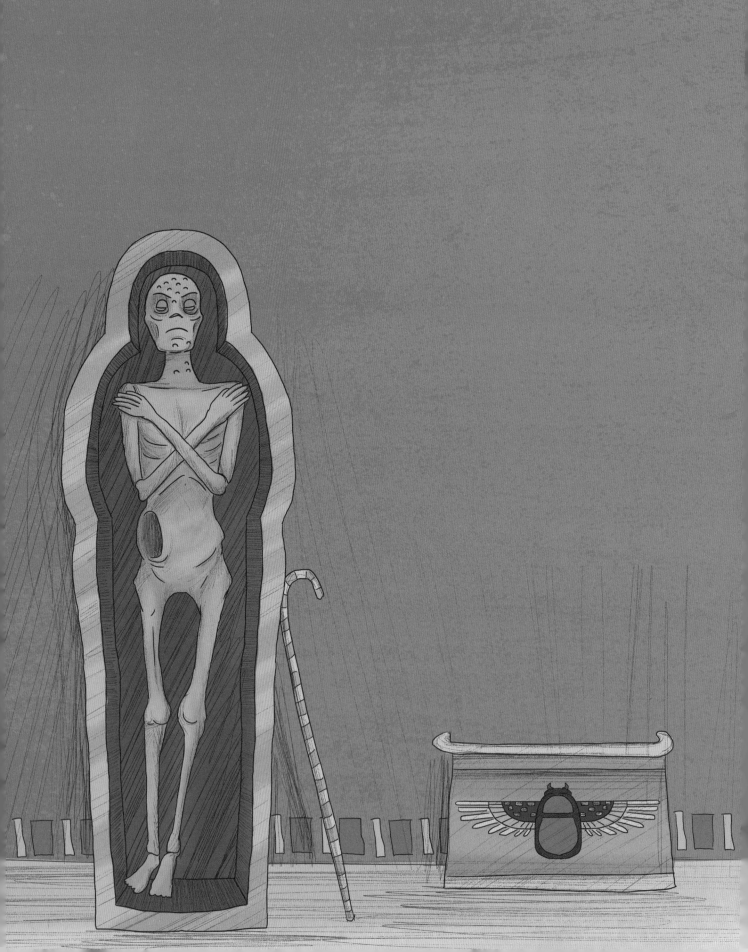

It's horrible having a fever, feeling sick and getting rashes, isn't it? But look inside this book and you'll witness the true horrors people faced in the past – rotting skin, damaged lungs, sinister pustules and swellings all over the body.

- The Black Death wiped out whole towns and villages
- Tuberculosis consumed young people like a blood-sucking vampire
- Smallpox left its victims scarred for life – if they survived ...

No one knew where these killer diseases came from or how to treat them. Frightening! See how people tried to ward them off and made vital discoveries. The Egyptians chewed garlic to keep malaria at bay, an English physician found the source of cholera, and a Cuban doctor showed that mosquitoes spread yellow fever – all pieces in the giant jigsaw puzzle of modern medicine.

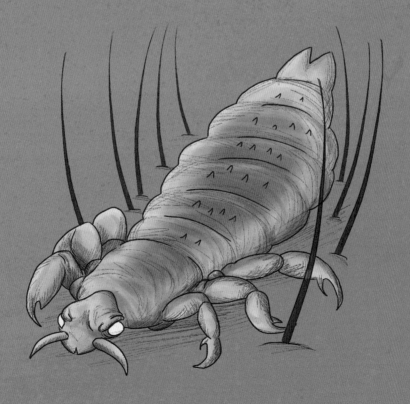

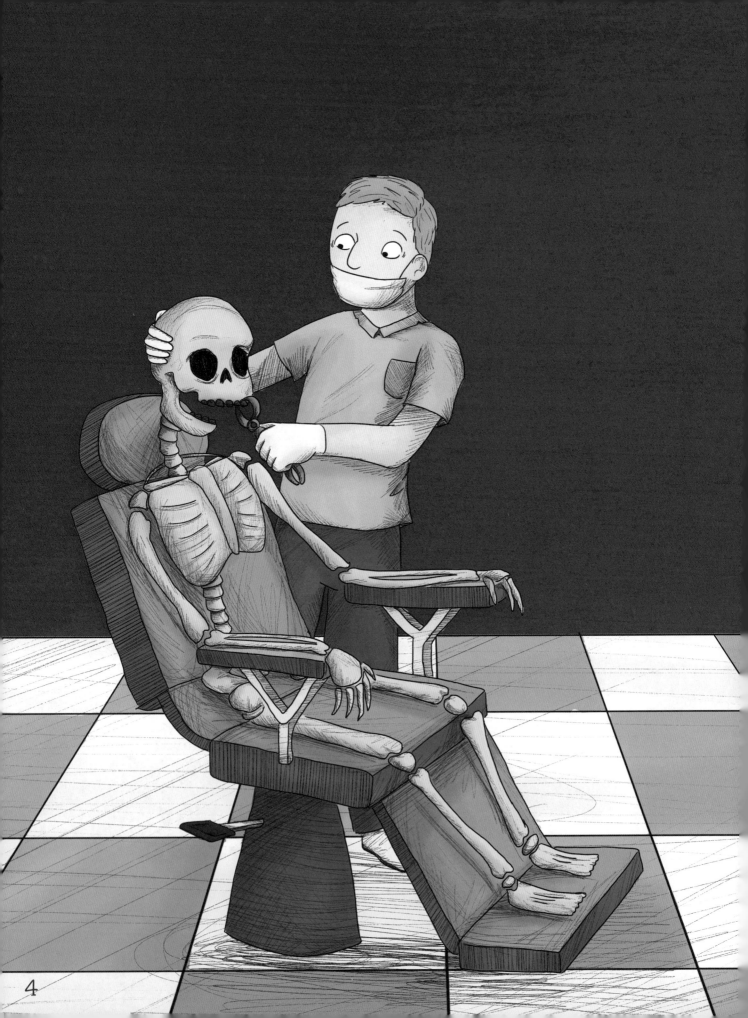

Contents

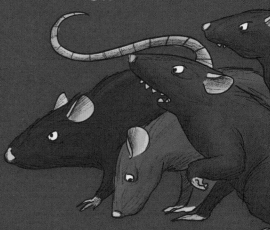

INTRODUCTION

It's not nice when you get sick. But if you ever feel sorry for yourself, then this book might just make you feel a little better. In the past, people were battered again and again by horrible diseases that made their skin rot, their hair fall out, their hands turn black, their lungs collapse and their faces erupt with boils – and that's if they were lucky...

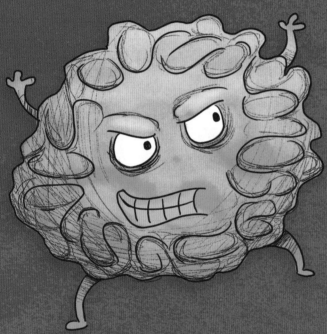

A happy ending

Smallpox made life utterly dreadful for English children in the 1700s. Only one out of every three children under the age of three survived it. But smallpox is one of the success stories of modern medicine. Thanks to the discovery of vaccination, it has vanished from the world entirely.

God's vengeance

One of the frightening things about diseases in the past is that people had no idea what caused them. Now we know diseases are spread by germs – tiny bacteria and viruses – so we can look for ways to fight them. But in the past there was no explanation. Many people simply believed diseases were caused by angry gods.

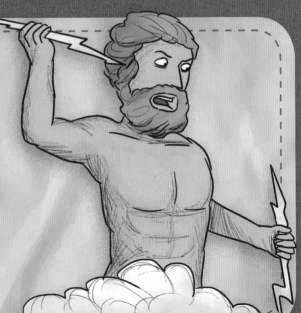

Deadly rider

In the past, diseases were so devastating that outbreaks were given frightening names, like 'plague' and 'pestilence'. These names are also given to one of the four horsemen of the apocalypse – four terrifying riders who will descend on the world on its final day of judgement, according to the Christian Bible.

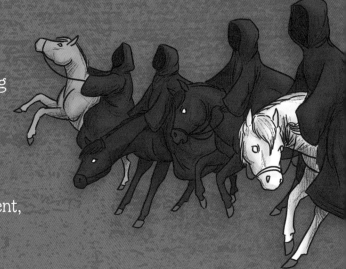

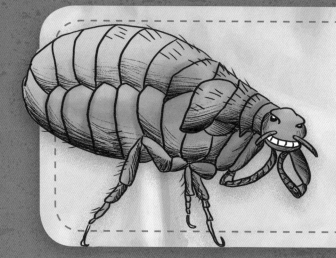

The outbreaks

Doctors today call the outbreaks of disease 'pandemics'. These spread far and wide, killing millions. Throughout history there have been many pandemics. One of the worst was the Black Death of 1347–1351, carried by fleas, which killed 25 million people in Europe.

It's the pits

It's hard to imagine just how bad outbreaks of disease were in the past. In many cities during the Black Death, there were too few people left to bury those who died. Bodies would be chucked into pits and left to rot.

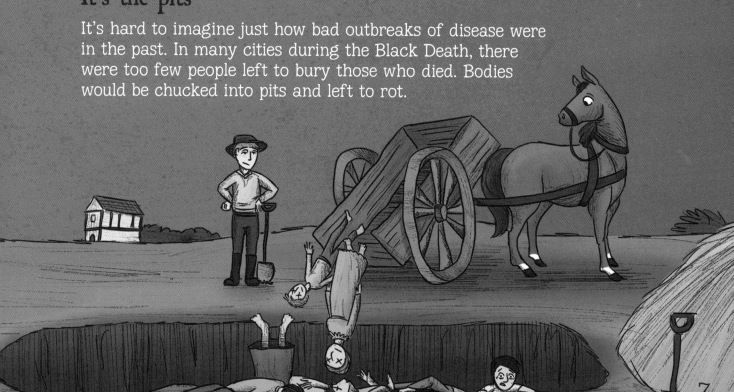

AN OLD KILLER

Malaria is a really terrible disease that affects mostly tropical regions. It kills nearly half a million people every year and makes over 200 million ill. People become infected when a mosquito bite injects a tiny microbe into their blood.

Tiny assassin

Malaria is caused by the microbe called *plasmodium*. But it is spread by female *Anopheles* mosquitoes. When this mosquito bites someone infected with the disease to feed on their blood, it picks up the microbe. When it bites someone else, it passes on the microbe, infecting them with malaria.

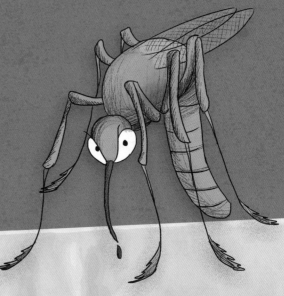

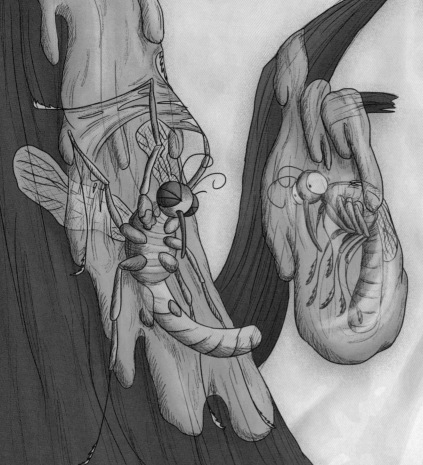

An ancient disease

Malaria is one of the oldest known diseases. The *plasmodium* microbes that cause it have been found in mosquitoes from as long ago as 30 million years. These mosquitoes were trapped in the resin that oozed from some trees, then perfectly preserved as the resin hardened and turned to amber.

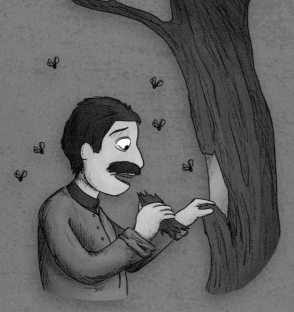

Fever tree

Malaria was spread to the Americas by European settlers in the 1500s. But the American Indians learnt to treat it using the powdered bark of the cinchona tree, which soon became known as the 'fever tree'. A drug called 'quinine', which is made from cinchona bark, is still an effective way of treating malaria.

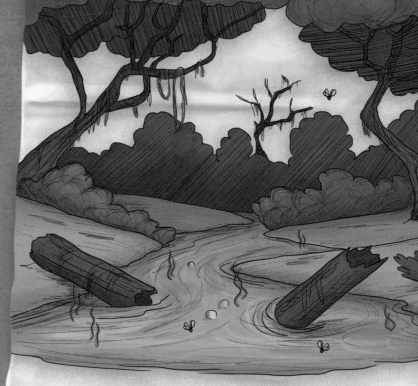

Bad air

The word 'malaria' comes from the Latin for 'bad air', and for a long time people thought it was caused by the damp, smelly air given off by swamps. They weren't so far wrong, because these swamps are the perfect breeding ground for the mosquitoes that pass on the disease.

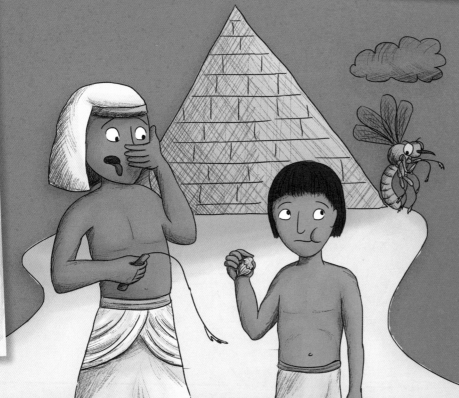

Smelly breath

Malaria became a killer disease as soon as people settled down to farm 10,000 years ago. The people who built the Egyptian pyramids stuffed themselves with garlic to ward off the disease. So they must have had very smelly breath! But scientists now think garlic really does help fight malaria.

9

DEADLY BLISTERS

In 541 AD –542 AD , the city of Constantinople (now Istanbul) was utterly ravaged by an outbreak of a terrible disease called the Justinian Plague, named after the city's ruler, Justinian. Up to 5,000 people died each day, and the streets were piled high with bodies.

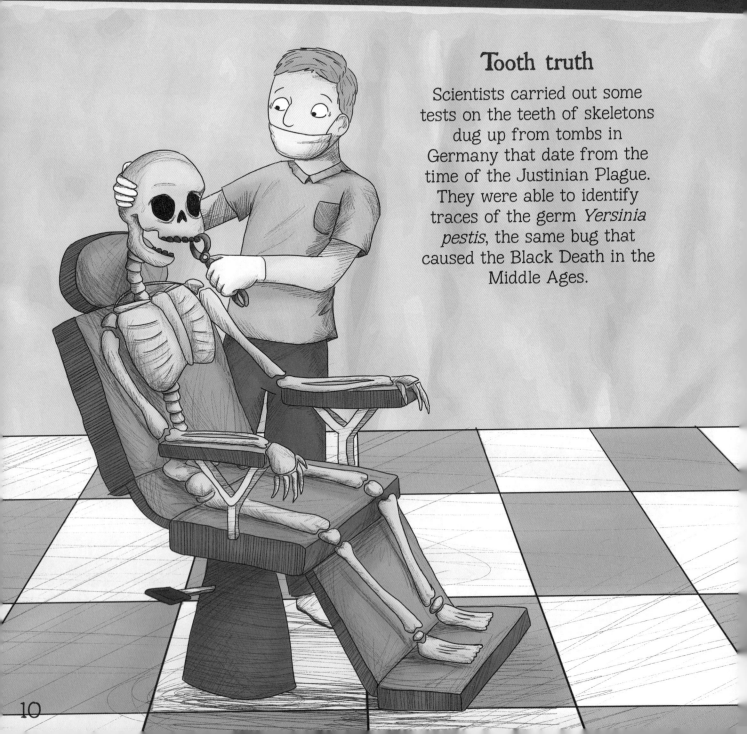

Tooth truth

Scientists carried out some tests on the teeth of skeletons dug up from tombs in Germany that date from the time of the Justinian Plague. They were able to identify traces of the germ *Yersinia pestis*, the same bug that caused the Black Death in the Middle Ages.

You look so well, ladies (not!)

If someone caught the plague, they would feel like they had the worst flu ever. Then parts of their body would turn black and their skin would erupt with terrible pus-filled swellings called 'buboes'. Within a week they'd be dead...

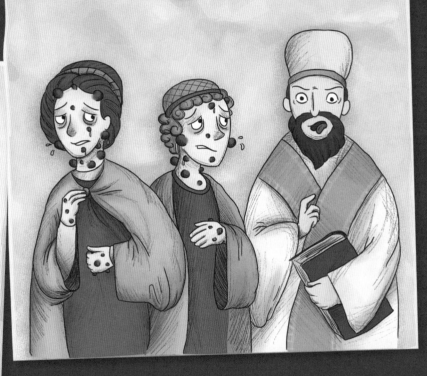

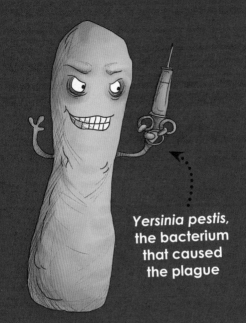

Yersinia pestis, the bacterium that caused the plague

That pesky *pestis*

Rats may have carried the disease to Constantinople, but the culprit was really a tiny bacterium called *Yersinia pestis*. *Yersinia pestis* may be tiny, but it was one of the deadliest killers in history. It also brought the Black Death in the Middle Ages, and the plague that killed millions in Asia in the later 1800s.

The march of death

The germs were carried to Constantinople by rats that stowed away on ships carrying grain from Egypt. From Constantinople, the plague spread rapidly, engulfing most of North Africa, the Middle East and Europe.

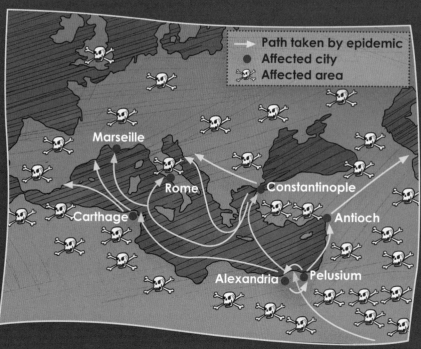

→ Path taken by epidemic
● Affected city
☠ Affected area

Marseille
Rome
Carthage
Constantinople
Antioch
Alexandria
Pelusium

THE BLACK DEATH

No disease has ever been quite so terrifying and deadly as the Black Death. It killed up to 25 million people in Europe between 1347 and 1351. In places, whole towns and villages were wiped out and there was no one left to bury the dead.

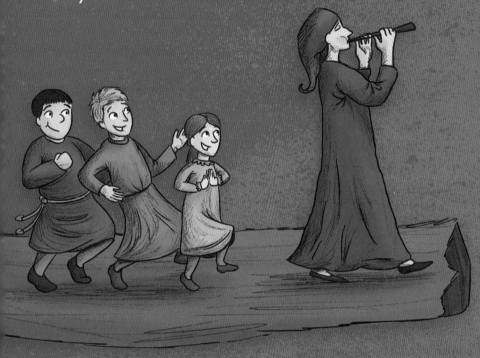

The Pied Piper

According to legend, the town of Hamelin in Germany was infested by rats. The town hired a piper who lured the rats out of the city to drown in the river and saved the city from the plague. But the mayor of the town, the legend says, failed to pay the piper for his work, so the piper lured the town's children away too...

Dance of death

After the plague, the shadow of death hung heavily over the people of the Middle Ages, and it became a key theme in art of the time. Many artists drew pictures of the 'danse macabre', or 'dance of death', in which the dead invited people from all walks of life to dance on a grave, showing how death comes to all.

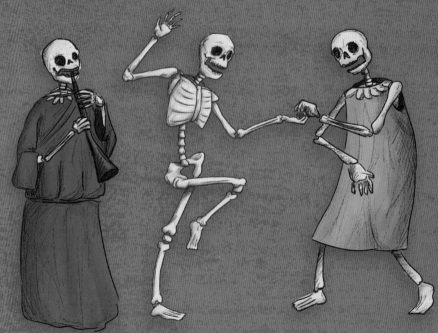

Mass burial

So many people died so quickly that the streets were piled with corpses, and the smell of rotting flesh was terrible. There were so many bodies to dispose of that the survivors just dug large trenches and piled them in one on top of the other, then covered them over with a little earth.

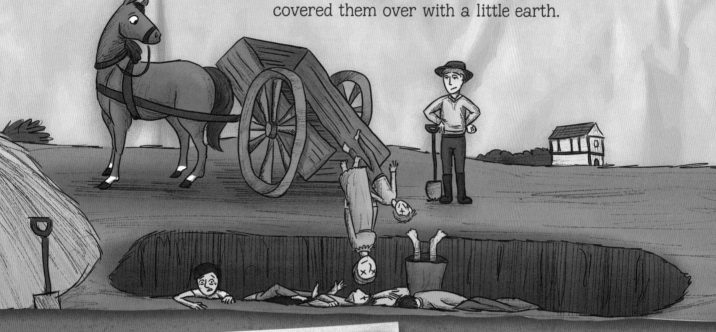

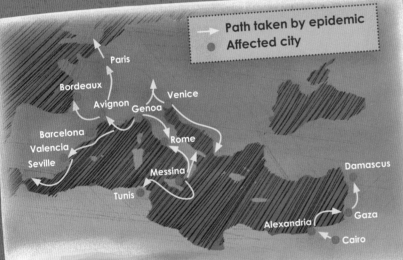

Path taken by epidemic
Affected city

Paris
Bordeaux
Avignon — Venice
Barcelona — Genoa
Valencia — Rome
Seville
Messina
Tunis
Damascus
Alexandria — Gaza
Cairo

Plague out of the East

The plague may have started in Central Asia and spread west. It reached Europe when Mongol armies catapulted infected corpses into the city of Kaffa in the Crimea as they besieged it in 1347. Genoese traders trapped in the city fled, carrying the infection with them to Europe.

Don't blame the rats

The Black Death was probably the bubonic plague, a horrible disease caused by the bacterium *Yersinia pestis*. In the 1600s people thought it was passed on to humans by black rats. But scientists now think the disease first came from gerbils, not rats.

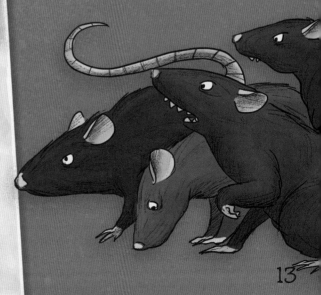

13

THE GREAT PLAGUE

The Black Death was thought to be the worst outbreak of disease in history. But for more than three centuries after it, Europe was subjected to repeated plagues. One massive outbreak was the 'Great Plague', which struck London in 1665.

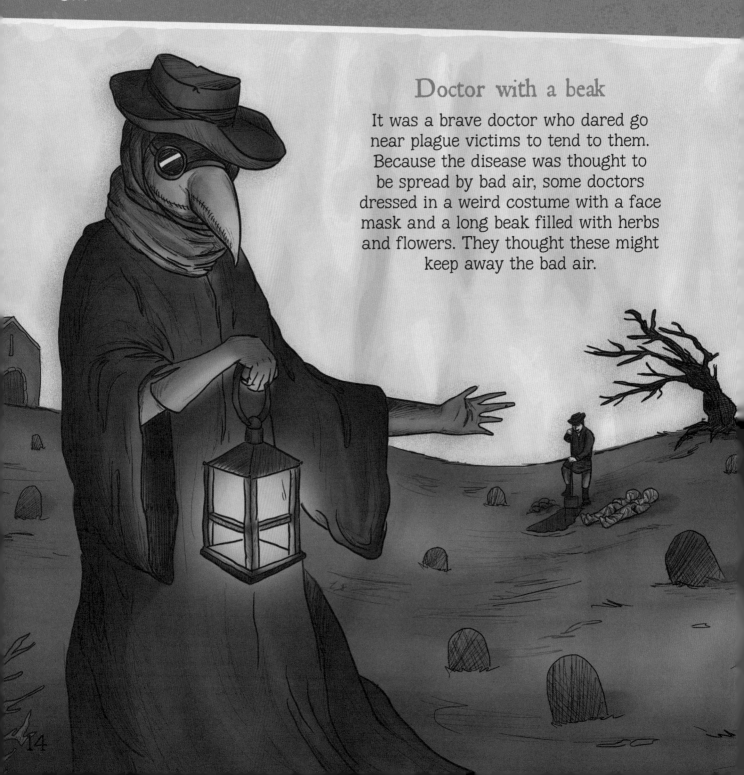

Doctor with a beak

It was a brave doctor who dared go near plague victims to tend to them. Because the disease was thought to be spread by bad air, some doctors dressed in a weird costume with a face mask and a long beak filled with herbs and flowers. They thought these might keep away the bad air.

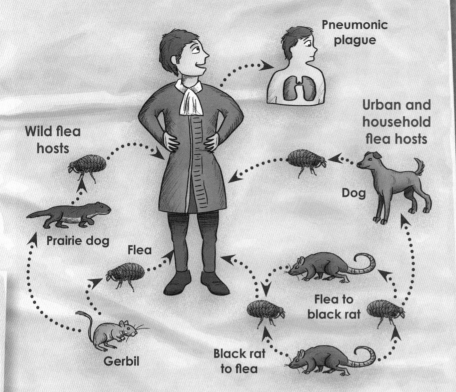

Pneumonic plague

Urban and household flea hosts

Dog

Wild flea hosts

Prairie dog

Flea

Gerbil

Black rat to flea

Flea to black rat

Plague pathway

Bubonic plague is caused by a bacterium that infects humans when they are bitten by a flea. These fleas live on rats. They can live on cats and dogs, too. Bubonic plague can then develop into pneumonic plague, which damages the lungs horribly and can be spread through the air in coughs and sneezes.

Little monsters

The *Yersinia pestis* bacterium that causes the bubonic plague is carried by fleas. But the pneumonic plague can be spread from one human to another through the air. The Black Death and Great Plague were probably a mix of both kinds.

Stinky streets

In the 17th century, there were no proper drains in cities like London, and people just chucked the contents of their toilets out into ditches in the narrow streets – often barely missing people walking past! In these filthy conditions, infections of all kinds could spread easily.

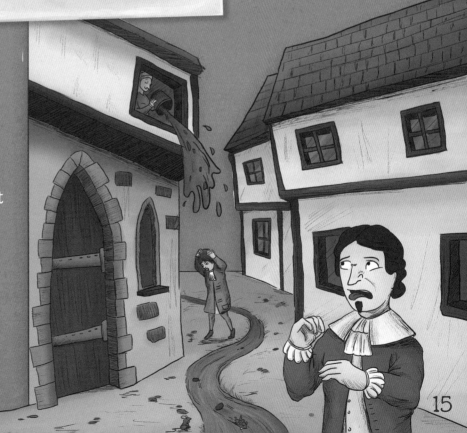

15

THE WHITE PLAGUE

Bubonic plague is now, thankfully, mostly a terror of the past. But the horrible lung disease tuberculosis, or TB, once known as the 'white plague', is still with us, and ten millions of people around the world are affected by it.

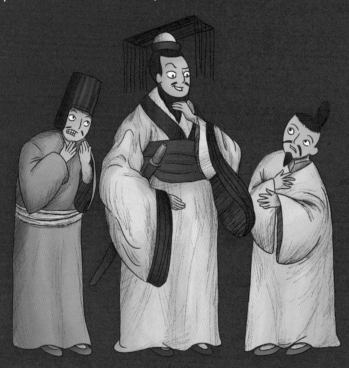

I'm an emperor and doctor

The mythical Chinese emperor, Huangdi (Yellow Emperor), has great contributions to Chinese medicine. A medical book called *Huangdi neijing*, said to be based on his ideas, contains the description of TB. It was written over 2,000 years after Huangdi's time.

Touch me, touch me!

TB doesn't just affect the lungs. It can cause swellings on the neck called 'scrofula'. In the Middle Ages, people with scrofula would queue up to see the king, because it was thought that being touched by the king would cure them. So the disease became known as the King's Evil.

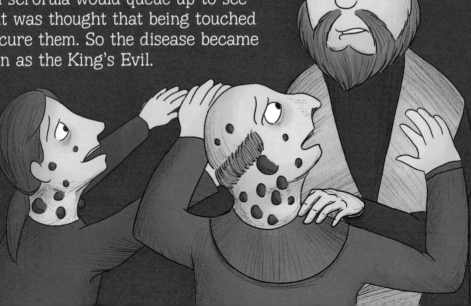

Symptoms of tuberculosis

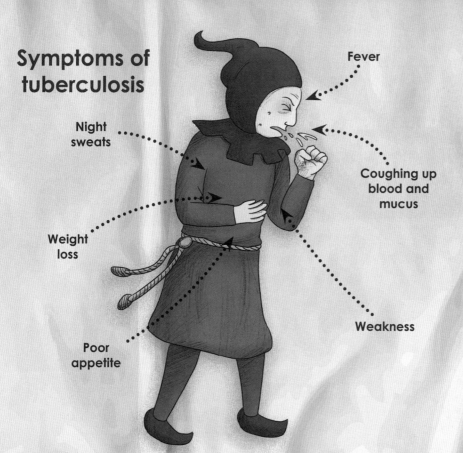

Fever

Night sweats

Coughing up blood and mucus

Weight loss

Weakness

Poor appetite

Coughs and fever

TB is a horrible disease that kills people slowly if they are not treated. It makes people cough terribly, often spitting up blood. It makes them sweat badly at night. And it makes them lose a lot of weight and become weak, which is why it came to be called 'consumption', because it seemed to consume the victim's body.

Vampire killers

People once thought TB victims had pale skin because vampires were sucking their blood and draining their lives away. That's why, when so many young girls died of consumption in the 1800s, writers wrote horror stories about vampire attacks.

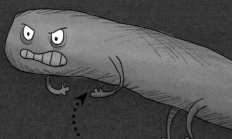

The *Mycobacterium tuberculosis* (MTB) bacterium, which causes TB

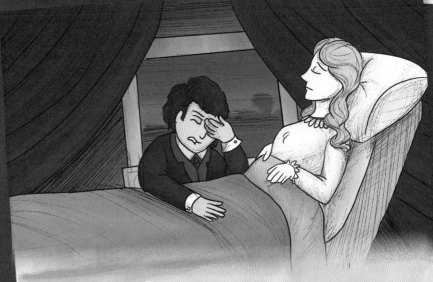

Romantic death?

In the 1800s, consumption claimed the lives of many young poets, such as John Keats, and many young girls. Their pale skin, for some, had 'a terrible beauty'. And so the disease came to seem almost romantic. But the victims suffered terribly, and their deaths caused their loved ones great heartache.

THE POX

Thanks to vaccination, the disease smallpox is dead. But for a long time in the past it was one of the world's worst killers, and even those who survived usually ended up with faces horribly disfigured by the skin rash it caused.

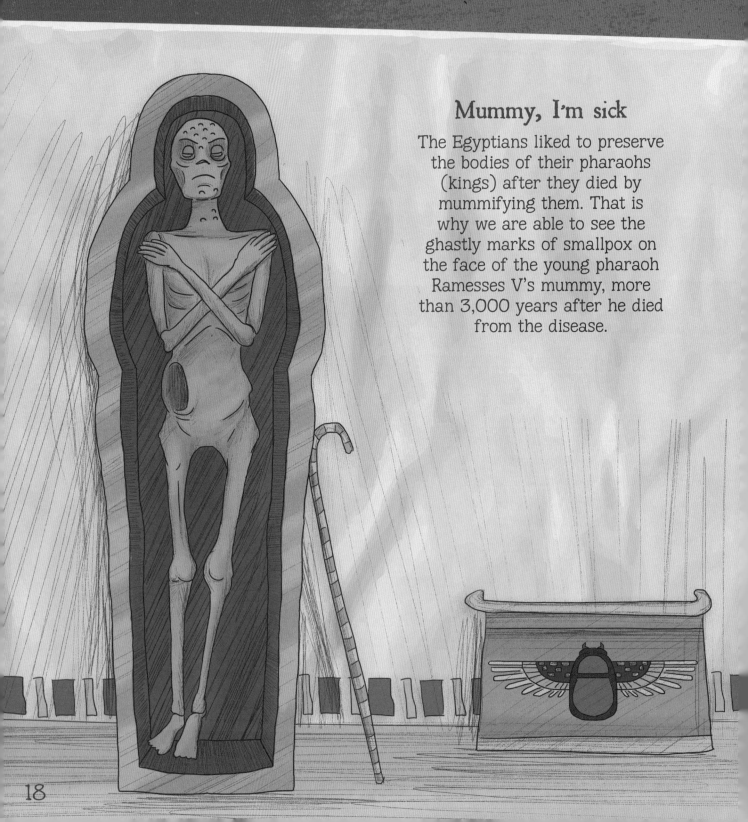

Mummy, I'm sick

The Egyptians liked to preserve the bodies of their pharaohs (kings) after they died by mummifying them. That is why we are able to see the ghastly marks of smallpox on the face of the young pharaoh Ramesses V's mummy, more than 3,000 years after he died from the disease.

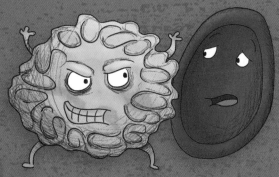

White queen

In October 1562, the young Elizabeth I of England caught smallpox. For a week her life hung in the balance. She pulled through, but her face was scarred by the disease and her hair fell out. For the rest of her life, she painted her face in thick white lead paint and egg whites, and wore wigs.

Nasty virus

Smallpox is caused by a virus called variola. It jumped from rodents to humans 16,000 years ago, and learnt how to invade body cells, causing smallpox. Thanks to vaccination, there are now just a few variola viruses left – safely locked up!

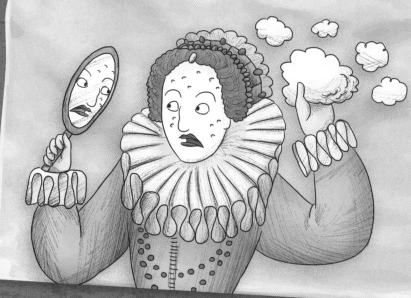

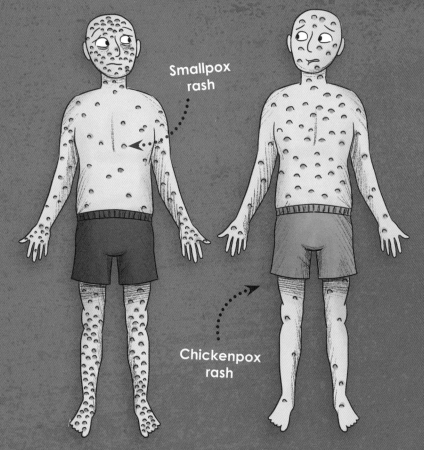

Smallpox rash

Chickenpox rash

Signs of smallpox

For two weeks after a person catches the smallpox virus, nothing happens. Then they start to feel like they have flu, but seem to get better. Suddenly red spots appear on their face and forearms, before spreading over their whole body and they become very ill. Smallpox can look like mild chickenpox, but the marks are much denser.

19

NAPOLEON'S NIGHTMARE

Like smallpox, typhus has been almost eradicated, thanks to vaccination. But like smallpox, typhus was once a deadly disease that brought a great deal of suffering and death. At first, victims suffered from an illness like flu, then developed a terrible rash over their whole body.

Beaten by a microbe

The French emperor Napoleon conquered most of Europe. But after reaching Moscow in 1812 and finding it abandoned, he decided to retreat. On the way back, through a bitter winter, more of his army was killed by typhus than by the armies of Russia.

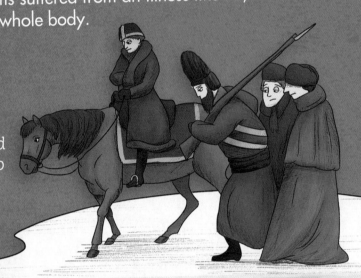

Nasty bugs

Typhus is caused by various kinds of bacteria called rickettsia. They infect humans via either animal droppings or nasty little lice or fleas. These can make people itch so much that they scratch their skin and make an opening for the bacteria.

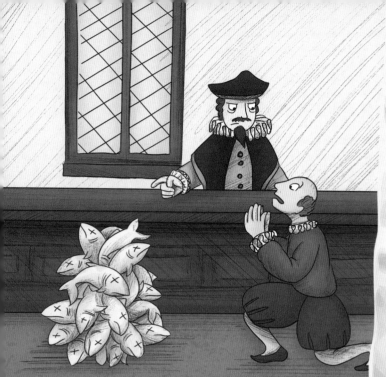

Delousing

In the aftermath of World War II, typhus could easily have spread rapidly among closely packed soldiers and the hordes of refugees. But millions of lives were saved when people were sprayed with the chemical, DDT, which killed the lice carrying the disease.

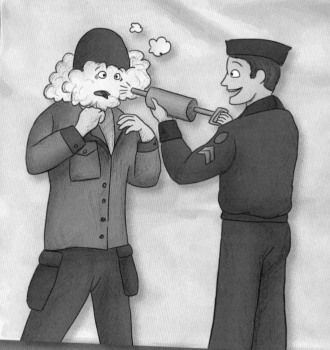

Sentenced to sickness

In the 1500s, many crime suspects died in prison of typhus or 'jail fever' before they could be tried. In 1586, 38 fishermen accused of stealing fish were carried into court in Exeter, England, half dead of typhus – and spread the disease to the court officials!

Irish fever

The poor in Ireland suffered especially from typhus at the time of the Irish famine in the 1840s. Many starved, and just as many were forced to leave their homes for other countries, when a disease killed off the potatoes that they relied on for food. From Ireland, typhus spread to England and became known as 'Irish fever'.

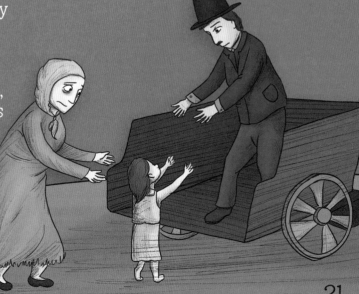

21

CHOLERA

Cholera is one of the nastiest diseases there is, giving people diarrhoea and making them horribly sick. People become infected by drinking dirty water in which the bacterium *Vibrio cholerae* thrives.

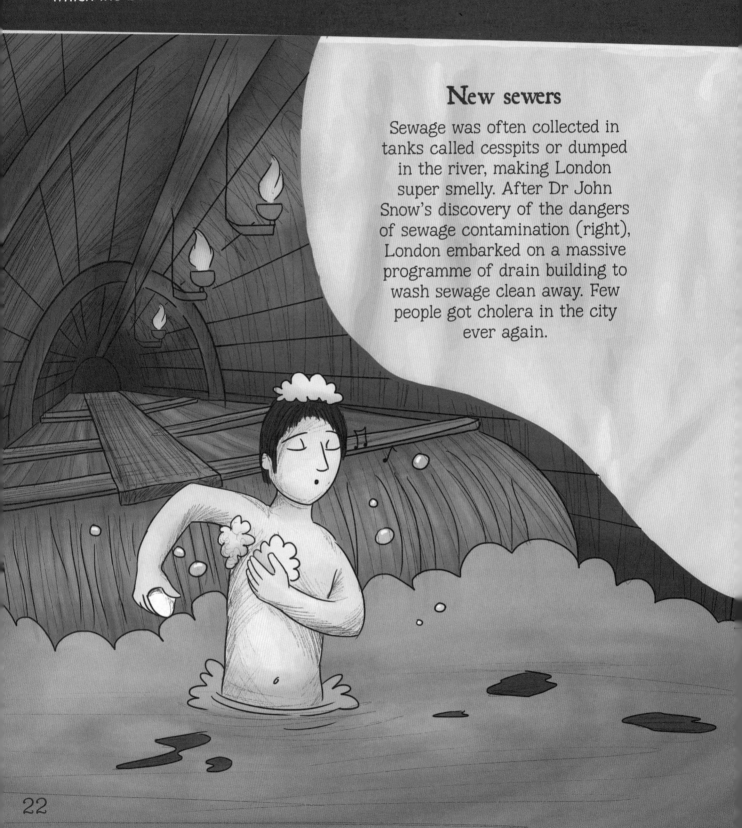

New sewers

Sewage was often collected in tanks called cesspits or dumped in the river, making London super smelly. After Dr John Snow's discovery of the dangers of sewage contamination (right), London embarked on a massive programme of drain building to wash sewage clean away. Few people got cholera in the city ever again.

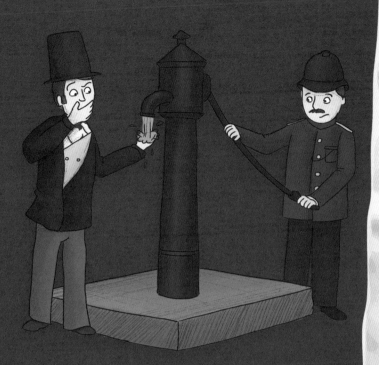

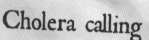

Cholera calling

The *Vibrio cholerae* bacterium that causes cholera thrives in water and food that has been contaminated by human poo. Humans can catch cholera if they eat sea creatures that swim in sewage-contaminated water. When people eat or drink anything containing cholera germs, they multiply in the gut and cause serious illness.

Snow's discovery

No one knew what caused cholera until an outbreak of the disease in London's Soho in 1854 prompted Dr John Snow to investigate. Snow found that victims had all drunk water from a pump in Broadwick Street. It turned out that the pump water was being contaminated by leaking sewage.

Flying the flag

Cholera became widespread in the 19th century when towns grew, yet people had poor access to clean water and poor sewerage systems. If anyone on board a ship came down with cholera, the ship had to fly a yellow-and-black flag to warn other ships. No one from the ship would be allowed ashore for a month.

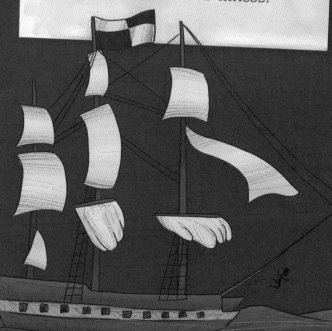

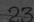

YELLOW FEVER

Yellow fever is a dangerous tropical disease that makes people very ill with fever and vomiting. Sometimes it makes the skin turn yellow as the germs damage the cells of the liver.

Yellow for danger

In most cases, yellow fever only makes people sweaty and sick for a few days. But for one in six people, the virus then attacks the liver, making the skin turn yellow and causing a nasty abdominal pain. Then the mouth and eyes bleed, and so does the gut, making the sufferer vomit black blood.

Symptoms of yellow fever

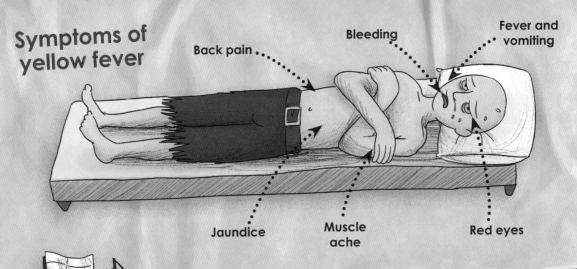

Back pain

Bleeding

Fever and vomiting

Jaundice

Muscle ache

Red eyes

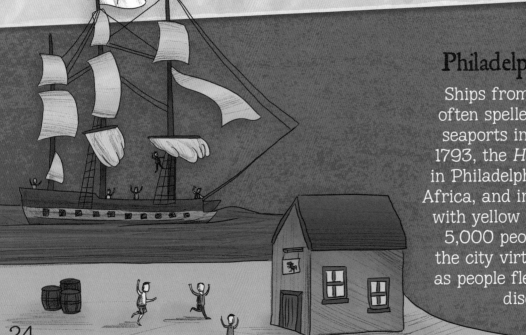

Philadelphia terror

Ships from the tropics often spelled trouble for seaports in the past. In 1793, the *Hanley* arrived in Philadelphia from West Africa, and infected the city with yellow fever. Around 5,000 people died and the city virtually emptied as people fled the terrible disease.

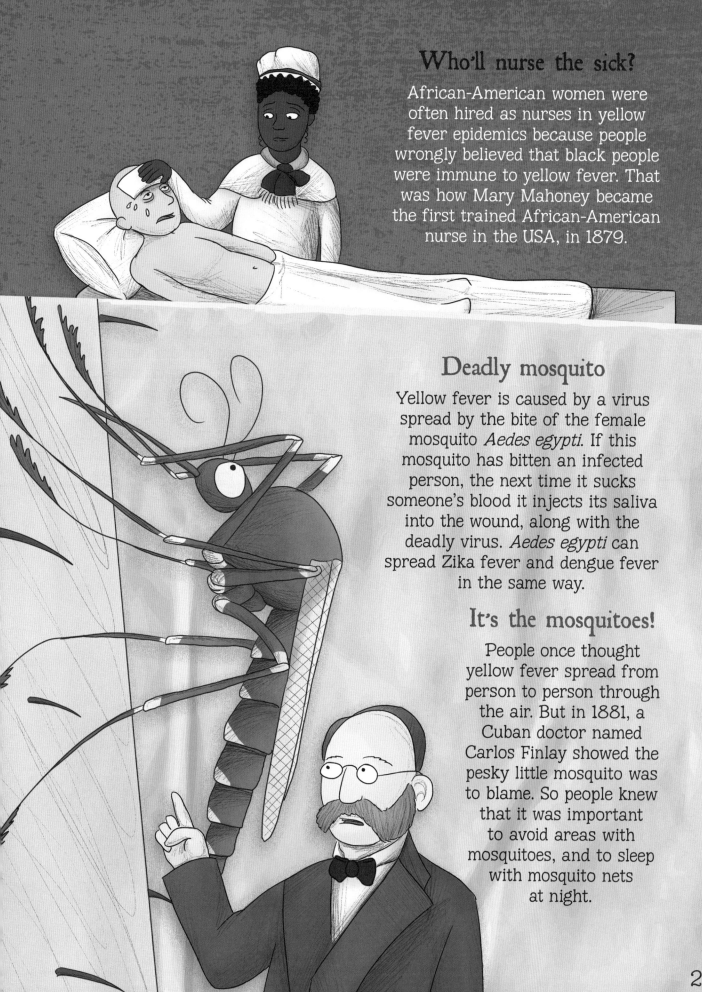

Who'll nurse the sick?

African-American women were often hired as nurses in yellow fever epidemics because people wrongly believed that black people were immune to yellow fever. That was how Mary Mahoney became the first trained African-American nurse in the USA, in 1879.

Deadly mosquito

Yellow fever is caused by a virus spread by the bite of the female mosquito *Aedes egypti*. If this mosquito has bitten an infected person, the next time it sucks someone's blood it injects its saliva into the wound, along with the deadly virus. *Aedes egypti* can spread Zika fever and dengue fever in the same way.

It's the mosquitoes!

People once thought yellow fever spread from person to person through the air. But in 1881, a Cuban doctor named Carlos Finlay showed the pesky little mosquito was to blame. So people knew that it was important to avoid areas with mosquitoes, and to sleep with mosquito nets at night.

SPANISH FLU

Most of the time, flu is just a minor winter illness. But some forms are deadly killers. An outbreak of one particular kind called 'Spanish flu' killed between 20 and 40 million people in 1918–1919, making it one of the deadliest disasters ever.

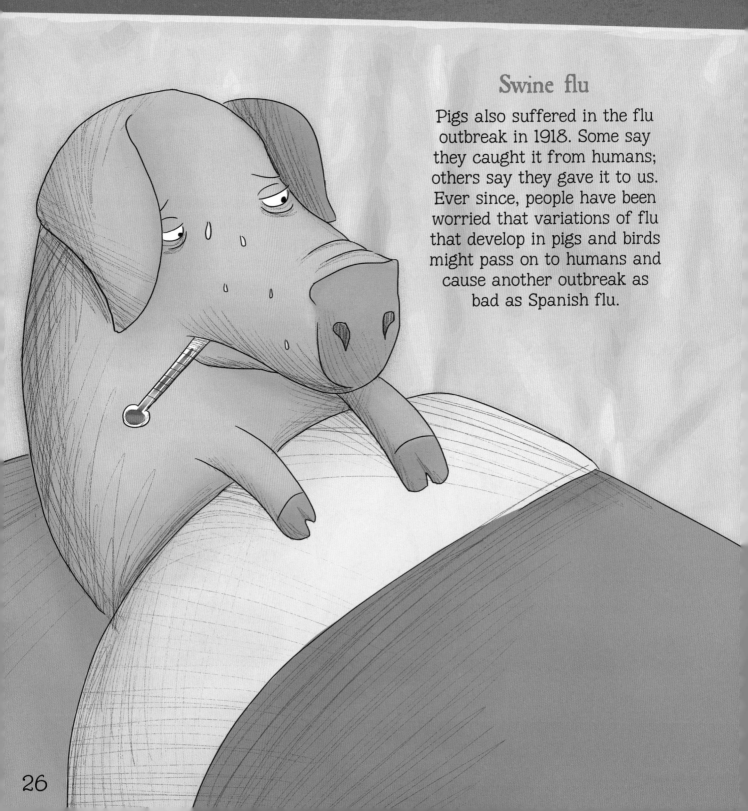

Swine flu

Pigs also suffered in the flu outbreak in 1918. Some say they caught it from humans; others say they gave it to us. Ever since, people have been worried that variations of flu that develop in pigs and birds might pass on to humans and cause another outbreak as bad as Spanish flu.

Flu in the trenches

In World War I, millions of soldiers were crowded together in muddy trenches in France. Pigs were crammed up near them, too, to provide food. It's thought the flu virus developed its deadly form as it was passed back and forth between pigs and soldiers.

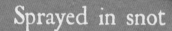

Sprayed in snot

Flu is very contagious, or easily spread. Someone with flu only has to sneeze for tiny droplets full of the virus to spray into the air and for someone else to breathe them in. During serious flu outbreaks, people may wear masks to avoid breathing in germs, but they are not very effective.

Camp Funston

Camp Funston might sound like a nice place to go on holiday. But in March 1918 it was anything but. It was a training camp for young soldiers in Kansas, USA, and is thought to be where the terrible Spanish flu epidemic began.

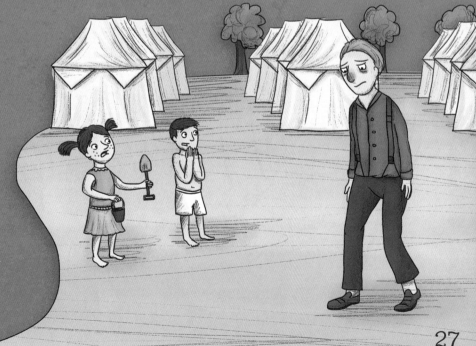

PESTILENTIAL TIMES

Thankfully most outbreaks of diseases come to an end – when they run out of victims, or victims recover. But they cause a lot of suffering. Here are some of history's worst.

541-542 AD
Justinian Plague

This plague (probably bubonic plague) spread out from Constantinople (modern Istanbul).

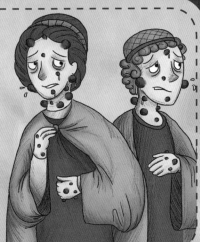

400 BC

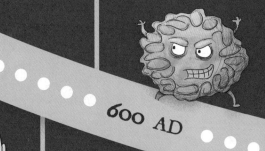

600 AD

430 BC
Plague of Athens

Ancient Athens was once very powerful – until it was hit by a terrible outbreak of disease, which experts believe may have been typhus but are not sure.

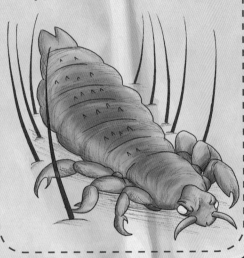

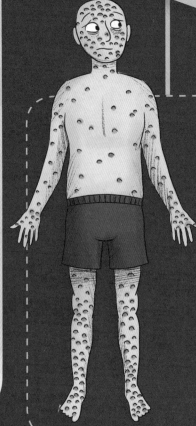

165-180 AD
Antonine Plague

In 165 AD the Roman Empire was ravaged by a pandemic that killed 5 million people, and fatally weakened the power of Rome. Experts now think it might have been smallpox or measles.

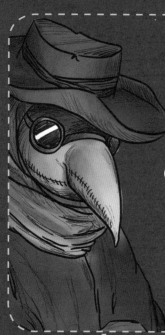

1665-1666
Great Plague of London

The plague kept coming back, but the Great Plague was the last major outbreak in Europe, killing 100,000 people in London – a quarter of the city's entire population.

1918-1919 Spanish flu

Immediately after World War I, the world was hit by one of the worst ever outbreaks of flu, called the Spanish flu. It infected one fifth of the population around the world and killed up to 40 million.

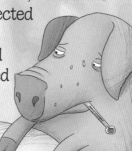

1855 Third Plague

Following the Justinian Plague and the Black Death, there was a third great pandemic of plague. It largely began in China in 1855 and swept through India to reach the Americas.

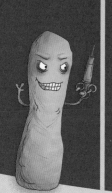

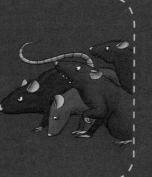

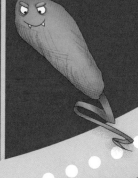

1700

1900

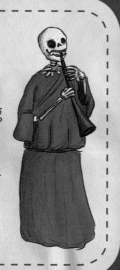

1347-1351
Black Death

This was one of the most terrifying pandemics ever. It killed 25 million people in Europe – a third of the population – in just several years.

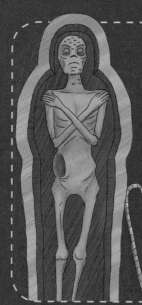

20th century Smallpox

Before it was finally eradicated in 1980, smallpox killed many people in the world during the 20th century, so it was perhaps one of the worst killers ever. Thank goodness it is no more!

GRUESOME SYMPTOMS

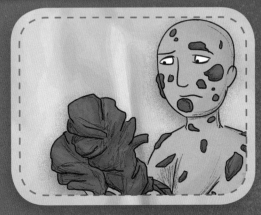

Epidermodysplasia verruciformis is a very rare disease that makes giant warts grow thickly all over the body.

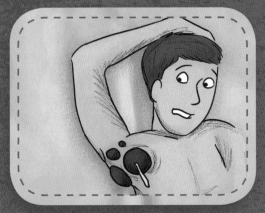

Buboes are horrible pus-filled blisters that erupt under the arms or on the neck or groin. They are a sign of bubonic plague.

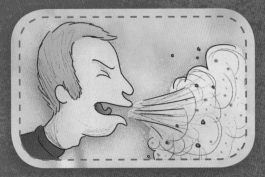

A single sneeze can spray out 6 million little viruses into the world.

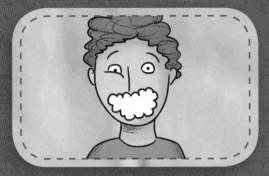

If a person were bitten by a dog with rabies, they might start dribbling and foaming at the mouth with saliva.

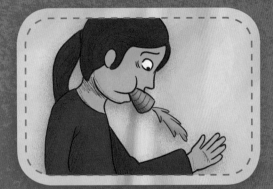

If someone throws up, their vomit often seems to contain carrots, even though they haven't eaten any! These are actually parts of the stomach lining that have come off.

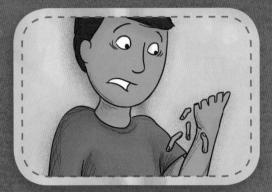

Leprosy has such horrific effects on the body, making bits drop off, that people suffering from the disease were once cut off from other people and forced to live in 'leper colonies'.

GLOSSARY

Amber	The resin that oozed from trees long ago and has turned solid
Bacterium	(plural: bacteria) A microbe made from just one cell
Black Death	The terrible pandemic of bubonic plague that swept through the world in the later 1340s, killing millions
Bubonic plague	A dreadful disease caused by the bacterium *Yersinia pestis* that often leads to distinctive buboes
Consumption	The old name for the killer lung disease named tuberculosis
Malaria	A tropical disease spread by one kind of mosquitoes
Microbe	An extremely small living thing which you can only see if you use a microscope
Mosquito	A tiny blood-sucking insect that can spread diseases such as malaria and yellow fever
Pandemic	A huge worldwide outbreak of an infectious disease
Plasmodium	A tiny organism that causes the disease malaria
Pneumonic plague	A dreadful disease related to bubonic plague that affects the lungs rather than causing buboes
Vaccination	The method of using dead or weakened germs to stimulate the body's immune system to guard against infection
White plague	A disease that makes the skin pale – usually tuberculosis

Index

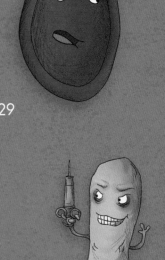

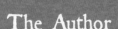

The Author

John Farndon is the author of many books on science, technology and nature, including the international best-sellers *Do Not Open* and *Do You Think You're Clever?* He has been shortlisted five times for the Royal Society's Young People's Book Prize.

The Illustrator

Venitia Dean grew up in Brighton, UK. She has loved drawing ever since she could hold a pencil. After receiving a digital drawing tablet for her 19th birthday she transferred to working digitally. She hasn't looked back since!

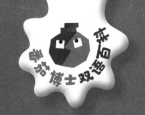

怪诞医学史

可怕的瘟疫

约翰·法恩登（英）著

温妮莎·迪安（英）绘

罗来鸥 译

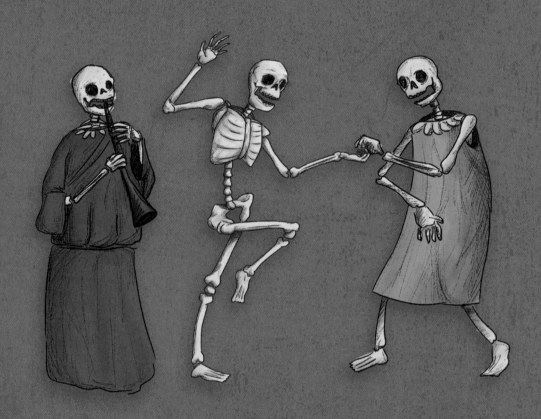

外语教学与研究出版社
FOREIGN LANGUAGE TEACHING AND RESEARCH PRESS
北京　BEIJING

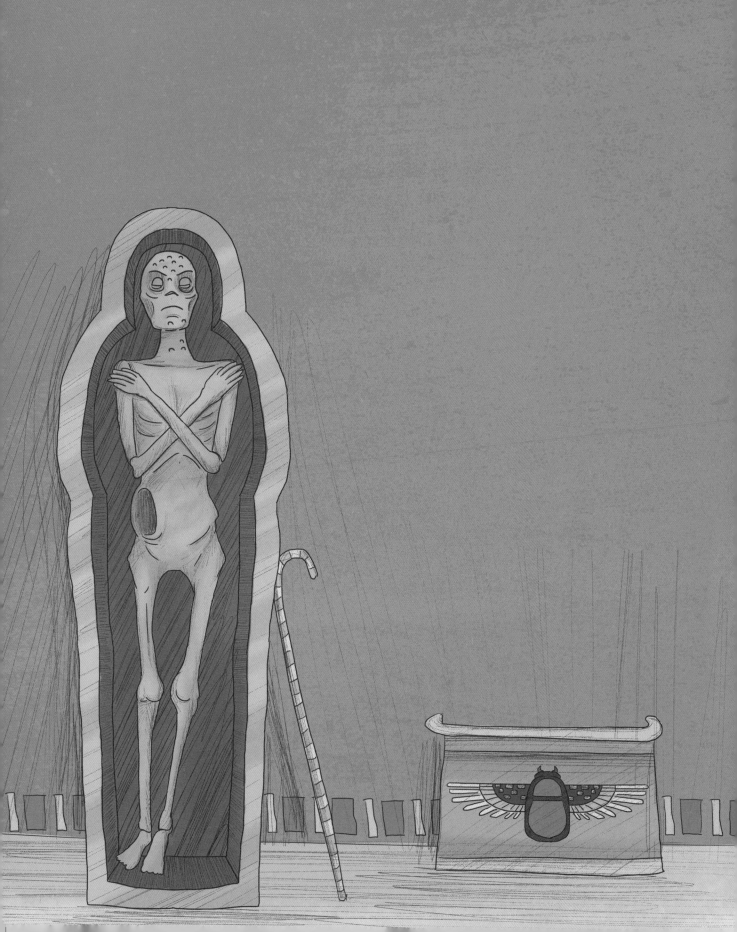

在生病时，发烧、恶心、身上出疹很难受，是不是？但是翻开这本书后，你会看到人们在过去面临的真正的恐怖——溃烂的皮肤、受损的肺部、恶性脓疱以及长满肿块的身体。

- 黑死病席卷了整座城镇和村庄
- 结核病像吸血鬼一样榨干年轻人
- 天花给幸存者留下终身的疤痕
  ……

当时没有人知道这些致命的疾病从何而来，又如何治疗。人们对病魔备感恐惧。但通过这本书，我们能看到人们如何设法击退疾病，并在与病魔抗争时取得了重大发现。埃及人通过咀嚼大蒜预防疟疾，英格兰医生找到了霍乱的根源，古巴医生发现了传播黄热病的元凶是蚊子——所有的这些都是现代医学大拼图中不可或缺的部分。

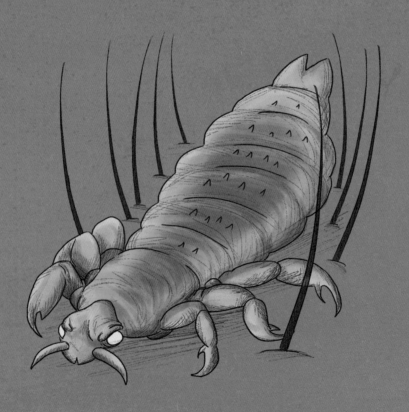

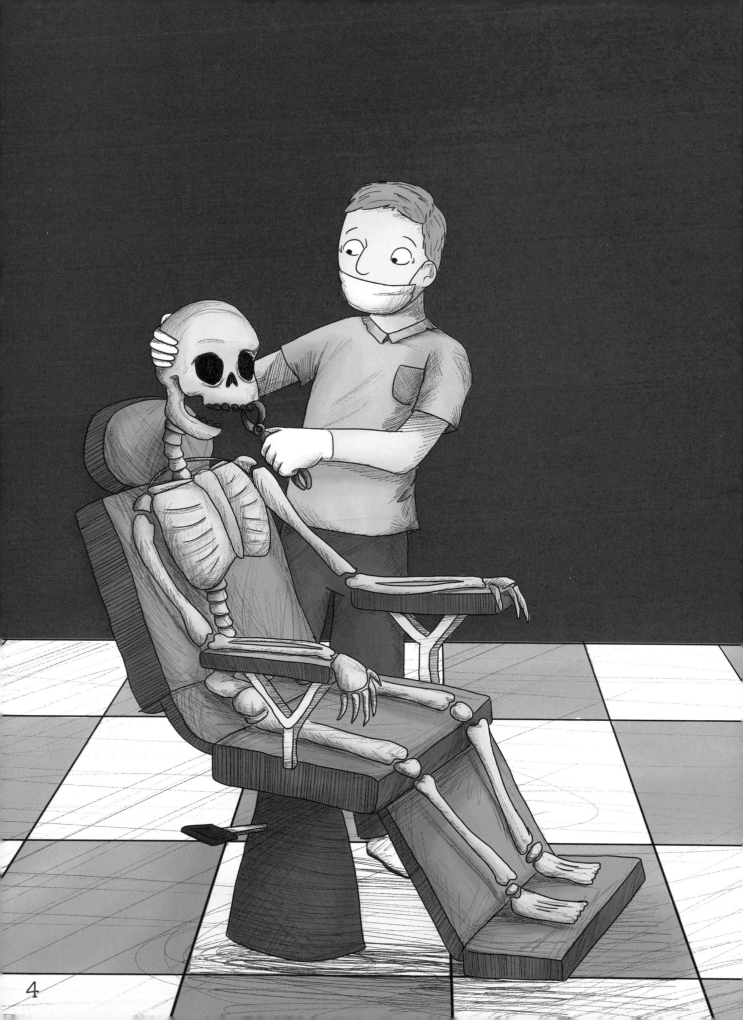

目录

写在前面

生病不是一件愉快的事。但如果你为自己生病而难过，那这本书也许会让你好受些。过去，人们被可怕的疾病反复折磨，他们患病后皮肤溃烂、头发脱落、双手黑青、肺部萎陷、满脸生疮，而这些人还算是幸运的……

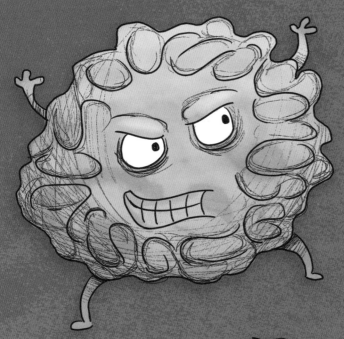

喜送瘟神

在18世纪，天花的流行使英格兰儿童在小小年纪便要经受生死考验。当时三岁以下染上天花的孩子中，只有三分之一能够活下来。而现代医学的一大贡献就是在天花防治上的突破。由于疫苗接种的出现和应用，天花已经从世界上彻底消失。

上天降祸论

过去，疾病如此可怕的一个原因是人们对它的成因一无所知。如今，我们知道疾病是由病菌——微小的细菌和病毒——传播的，这样我们就可以想办法对抗疾病。而过去人们找不到对疾病的合理解释，很多人就直接把它归因于神灵的动怒。

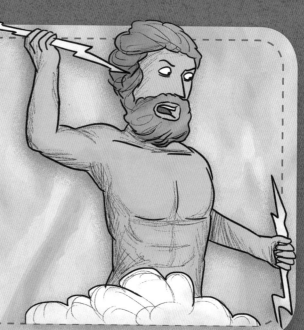

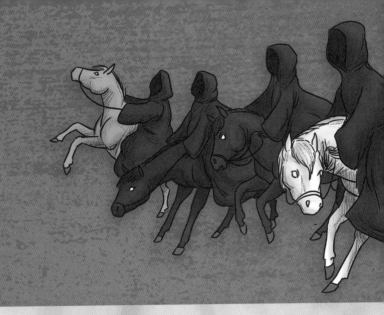

带来瘟疫的死亡骑士

过去医疗水平低下，疾病往往极具杀伤力，人们会给突然暴发的疾病起可怕的名字，如"瘟疫"或"疫病"。根据基督教《圣经》的说法，世界会迎来末日审判，恐怖的天启四骑士会在世界末日时降临于世，其中一个就叫"瘟疫"。

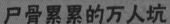

历史上的严重疫情

如今的医生把严重的疾病暴发事件称为"大流行病"。这些大流行病会在大片区域广泛传播，导致数以百万计的染病者丧命。人类历史上出现过很多次这样的大流行病，规模最大的疫情之一是1347年至1351年的黑死病。黑死病这种可怕的疾病由跳蚤传播，最终导致欧洲范围内2,500万人不治身亡。

尸骨累累的万人坑

很难想象过去疾病暴发时的情景有多恐怖。在黑死病暴发期间，大批城市居民死亡，侥幸存活的人太少，几乎找不到人去填埋死尸。于是，病死者的遗体被草草丢弃到大坑里，尸骨暴露在空气中，腐烂发臭。

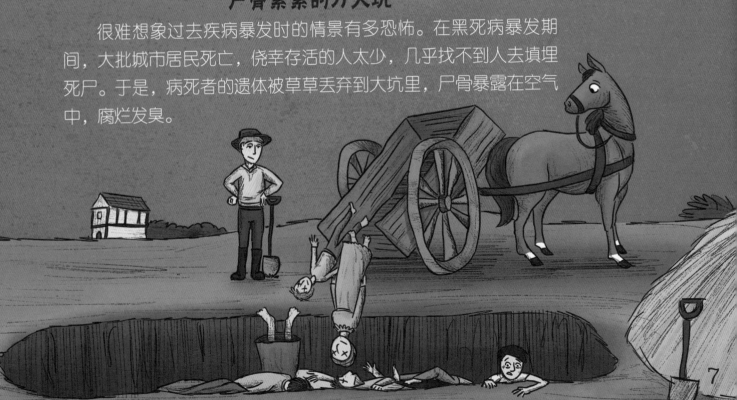

7

古老的顽疾：疟疾

疟疾是一种十分可怕的疾病，主要在热带地区流行。每年都会有近50万人死于疟疾，感染疟疾的人数更是超过两亿。疟疾通常是由一种蚊子传播，人们被这种蚊子叮咬后致病微生物就会被注入血液中。

不起眼的"刺客"：按蚊

疟疾的致病元凶是一种叫作疟原虫的微生物，而充当传播媒介的则是一种雌性按蚊。当这种蚊子叮咬疟疾患者以吸食血液时，也将疟原虫吸入体内。当它再叮咬其他人时就会传播疟原虫，导致其他人也感染疟疾。

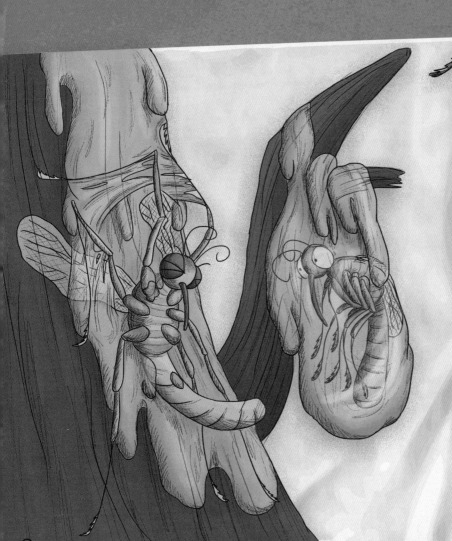

古老的疾病

疟疾是人类已知最古老的疾病之一。研究人员在3,000万年前的蚊子体内发现了疟原虫。这些蚊子被困在某些树木分泌的树脂中，在树脂硬化变为琥珀后，尸体就被完好地保存下来。

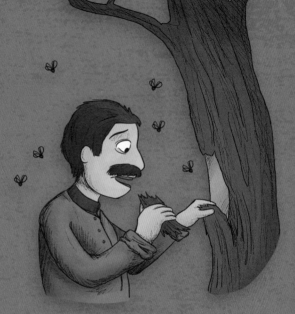

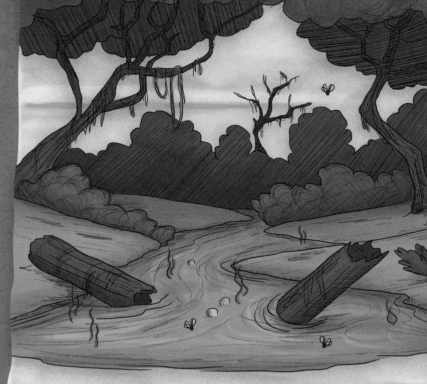

退热奇树：金鸡纳树

16世纪，欧洲殖民者把疟疾传到了美洲。但美洲印第安人摸索出了治疗疟疾的方法——服用研磨成粉末的金鸡纳树树皮。金鸡纳树很快被众人得知，得名"退热奇树"。而从金鸡纳树的树皮中提取的"奎宁"，直到现在仍然是一种有效的抗疟药。

臭气、沼泽与疟疾

"疟疾"的英文malaria源自拉丁语，意思是"浊气"。曾有很长一段时期，人们都认为是沼泽地里散发出的难闻湿气引发了疟疾。其实这种观点也不算太离谱，因为这样的沼泽地最易滋生传播疟疾的蚊子。

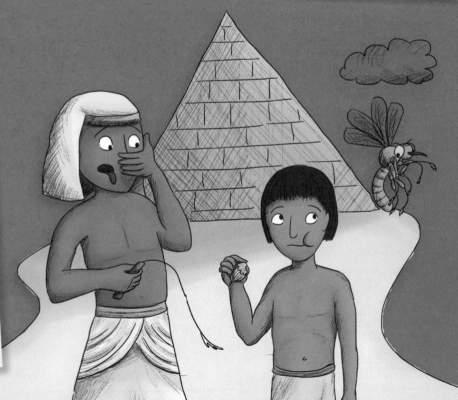

大蒜难闻，但能驱病

一万年前，当人们为了农耕而定居时，疟疾就成为导致人们丧命的可怕疾病。古埃及建造金字塔的劳工们靠往嘴里塞大蒜来预防疟疾，想必他们的口气一定很难闻。但现在的科学家们认为，大蒜确实有助于预防疟疾。

水疱也致命：查士丁尼瘟疫

公元541—542年，恐怖疾病查士丁尼瘟疫的暴发使君士坦丁堡（现在的伊斯坦布尔）遭遇灭顶之灾。因瘟疫暴发时是拜占庭皇帝查士丁尼在位，因此此次瘟疫被后人称为查士丁尼瘟疫。在瘟疫流行期间，君士坦丁堡每天有多达五千人死亡，街道上到处都是堆得高高的死尸。

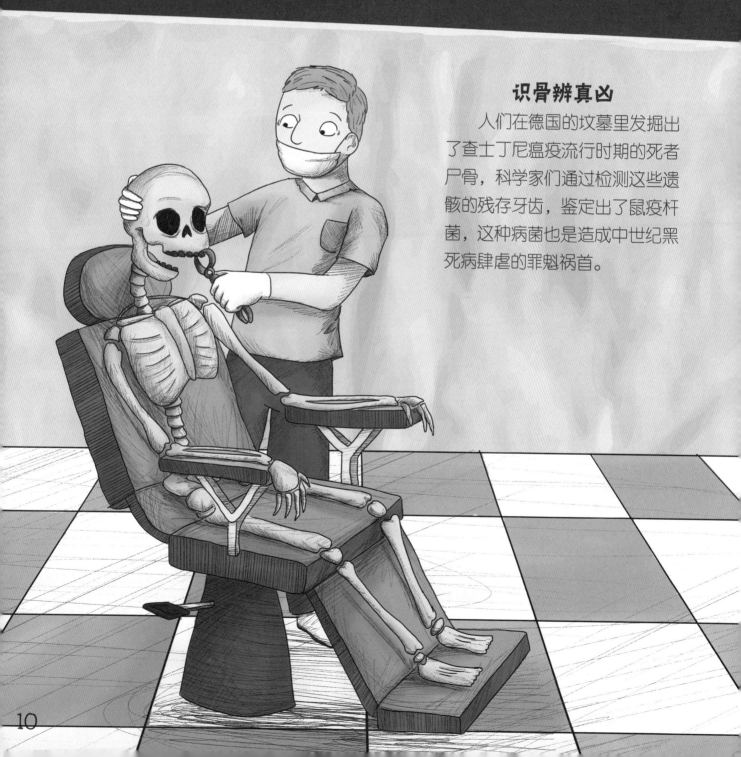

识骨辨真凶

人们在德国的坟墓里发掘出了查士丁尼瘟疫流行时期的死者尸骨，科学家们通过检测这些遗骸的残存牙齿，鉴定出了鼠疫杆菌，这种病菌也是造成中世纪黑死病肆虐的罪魁祸首。

花容月貌，转眼成灰

如果有人感染了查士丁尼瘟疫，他们起初会感觉像是患了最严重的流感。接下来，他们身体的一些部位会变黑，皮肤上长出充满脓液的可怕脓肿，也就是腹股沟淋巴结炎。患者在一星期之内就会死亡。

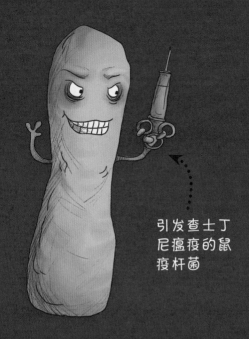

引发查士丁尼瘟疫的鼠疫杆菌

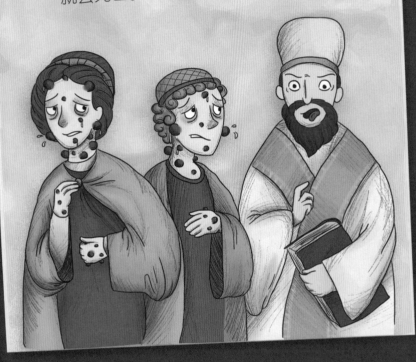

作恶多端的鼠疫杆菌

也许是老鼠把查士丁尼瘟疫传到了君士坦丁堡，但真凶其实是一种微小的细菌——鼠疫杆菌。鼠疫杆菌虽然小，在历史上却是最易致命的病菌之一。中世纪的黑死病就是它兴风作浪的结果，19世纪下半叶肆虐亚洲，夺去数百万人性命的瘟疫也是它的"杰作"。

瘟疫的远征

藏身于埃及运粮船里的老鼠将病菌带到了君士坦丁堡。疫情迅速从君士坦丁堡蔓延，北非大部分地区、中东及欧洲都沦为疫区。

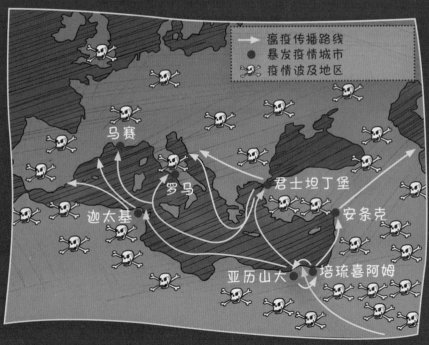

瘟疫传播路线
暴发疫情城市
疫情波及地区

马赛
罗马
迦太基
君士坦丁堡
安条克
亚历山大
培琉喜阿姆

死神的狂欢：黑死病降临

从古至今，没有哪种疾病像黑死病那样恐怖且致命。1347年至1351年，黑死病导致欧洲范围内多达2,500万的感染者命丧黄泉。在有些地区，整座城镇和村庄都被瘟疫吞噬，连埋葬死尸的人也找不到，因为没有人侥幸活下来。

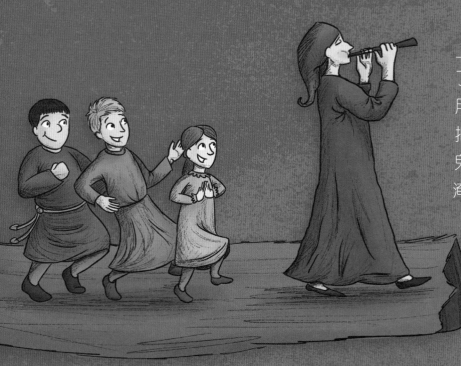

魔笛乐手的传说

传说中，德国哈梅林镇上的老鼠泛滥成灾。镇上雇了一个吹笛子的乐手，他能用笛子吹奏出魔幻的曲调，把老鼠们引出城外，让它们鬼使神差般地自己跳入河中淹死，从而使这座城市免遭黑死病的侵袭。可是，那个镇长没有付给乐手酬劳，于是这个乐手吹着笛子把镇上的孩子们也拐走了……

勾魂夺命的亡灵之舞

黑死病过后，死亡的阴影长久萦绕在中世纪人们的心中，死亡也成为那个时代艺术创作的主要题材。许多画家创作了关于"骷髅之舞"的画作，在画中，亡灵邀请各行各业的人们在墓地跳舞，意味着死亡所到之处，无人能够幸免。

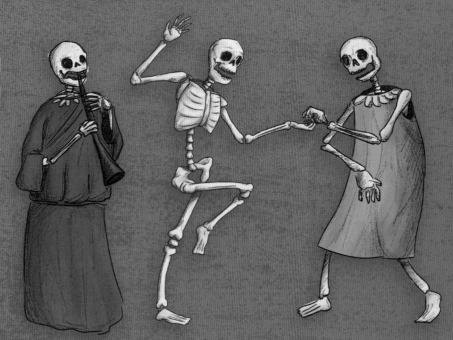

凄凉葬身万人坑

许多人染上黑死病后很快就死了，以至于城市的街道上堆满了尸体，空气中弥漫着呛人的腐尸气味。因为有太多的尸体需要处理，幸存者只好挖一些大坑，把尸体横七竖八地堆放在坑中，再盖上一层薄薄的土。

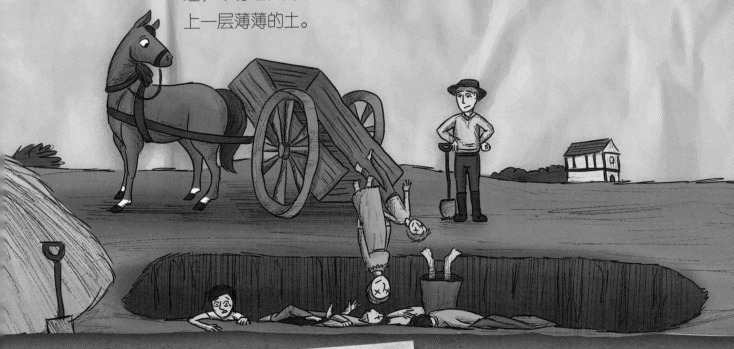

"背黑锅"的普通老鼠

黑死病很可能就是腺鼠疫，它是一种由鼠疫杆菌引发的可怕疾病。17世纪的时候，人们认为鼠疫杆菌是由普通黑老鼠传给人类的。但今天的科学家们认为，黑死病最初应该是来源于沙鼠，而不是普通老鼠。

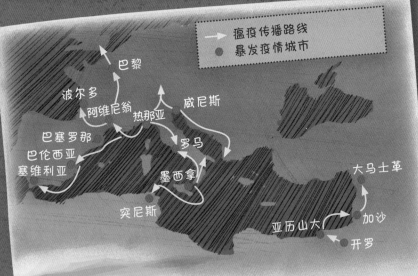

瘟疫传播路线
暴发疫情城市

巴黎
波尔多
阿维尼翁
热那亚
威尼斯
巴塞罗那
罗马
巴伦西亚
塞维利亚
墨西拿
突尼斯
大马士革
亚历山大
加沙
开罗

"恶魔"肆虐欧亚非

黑死病最早可能暴发于中亚地区，然后向西蔓延。1347年，蒙古军队在克里米亚半岛围攻卡法古城时，用投石机将黑死病患者的尸体投入城中。困在城里的热那亚商人伺机逃出城后，把黑死病带到了欧洲。

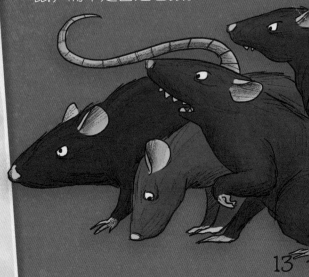

13

最后的疯狂：伦敦大瘟疫

有人认为黑死病是疾病传播史上最恐怖的一页。但在那以后的三个多世纪里，欧洲反复暴发了多次鼠疫，而其中一次大规模疫情于1665年在英国伦敦暴发，也就是"伦敦大瘟疫"。

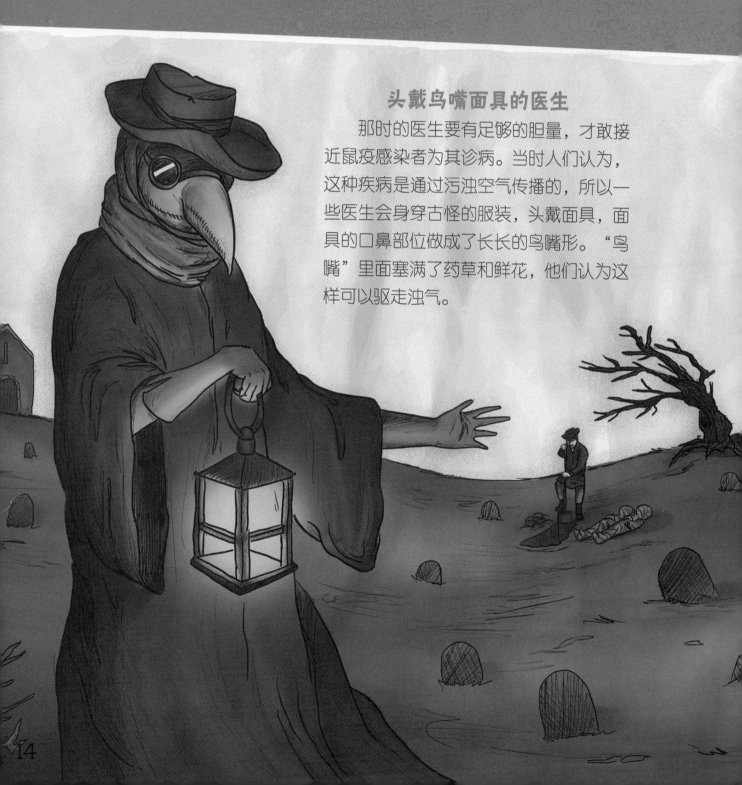

头戴鸟嘴面具的医生

那时的医生要有足够的胆量，才敢接近鼠疫感染者为其诊病。当时人们认为，这种疾病是通过污浊空气传播的，所以一些医生会身穿古怪的服装，头戴面具，面具的口鼻部位做成了长长的鸟嘴形。"鸟嘴"里面塞满了药草和鲜花，他们认为这样可以驱走浊气。

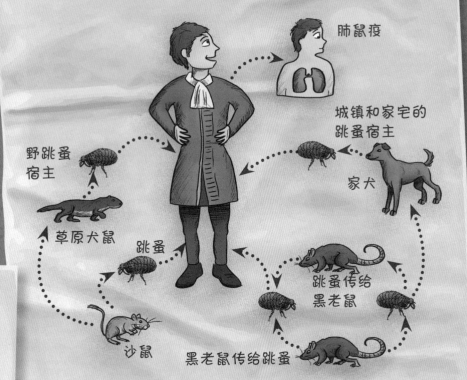

肺鼠疫

城镇和家宅的跳蚤宿主

野跳蚤宿主

家犬

草原犬鼠

跳蚤

跳蚤传给黑老鼠

沙鼠

黑老鼠传给跳蚤

鼠疫的传播途径

跳蚤通过叮咬把鼠疫杆菌传染给人类，继而引发腺鼠疫。这些跳蚤寄生在老鼠身上，也可以寄生在猫和狗身上。腺鼠疫有可能发展成肺鼠疫，严重损害肺部，并通过感染者咳出和喷出的空气传播给其他人。

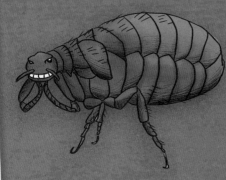

小小跳蚤惹灾殃

引发腺鼠疫的鼠疫杆菌是由跳蚤携带并传播的，但肺鼠疫却可以不经跳蚤直接由一个感染者通过空气传染给其他人。黑死病和伦敦大瘟疫很可能是这两种鼠疫同时传播的恶果。

臭气熏天的街巷

17世纪，像伦敦这样的大城市还没有完善的排污设施，人们把马桶中的粪便污物随意倾倒在狭窄街道的沟渠里，过往的路人往往差点就被泼溅上脏臭屎尿。这样肮脏不堪的环境很容易传播各种疾病。

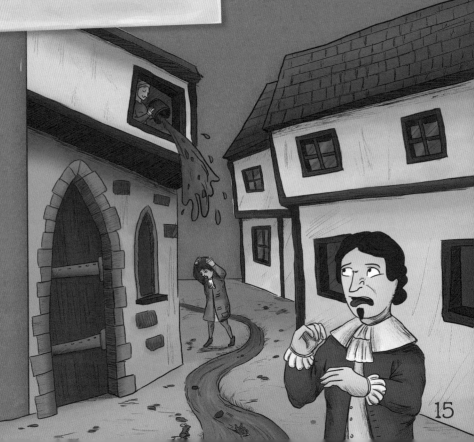

梦魇般的白色瘟疫：
结核病

　　谢天谢地，令人谈虎色变的腺鼠疫已基本成为过去了。然而，另外一种可怕的肺部疾病——结核病——直至今天仍然在威胁人类的健康，这种传染病曾经被人们称为"白色瘟疫"，如今全世界仍然有数千万人感染结核病。

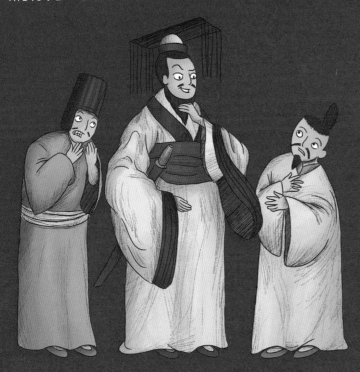

"皇帝医生"的卓越贡献

　　传说中的中国首领——黄帝，对中国医学有着巨大的贡献。据说，中国的医学典籍《黄帝内经》就是以黄帝的医学思想为基础编写的，书中包含对结核病的记载。但实际上，《黄帝内经》成书于黄帝去世两千多年以后。

"陛下救命！"

　　结核病不仅感染肺部，还会使人颈部出现肿块，即瘰疬（又称淋巴结结核）。中世纪时，那些受瘰疬折磨的患者会排队求见国王，因为当时人们认为被国王触碰便可以治愈这种病症，所以这种病又被称为"国王病"。

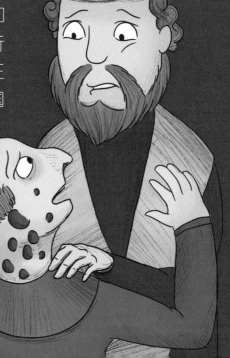

结核病的症状

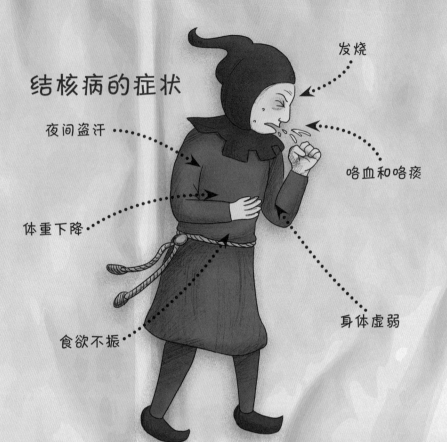

发烧

夜间盗汗

体重下降

食欲不振

咯血和咯痰

身体虚弱

咳嗽、咯血和发烧

结核病是一种非常可怕的疾病，如果不治疗，患病者会慢慢死去。结核病患者会咳嗽得非常厉害，常伴随咯血，夜间大汗淋漓。患者体重大幅下降，身体越来越虚弱。所以结核病又被称为"痨病"，因为它好似把患者的身体慢慢掏空。

吸血鬼的攻击

过去人们认为，结核病患者皮肤惨白是由于吸血鬼在吸他们的血，而他们的血被吸干后就会慢慢死去。因此在19世纪，当许多年轻女孩死于这种痨病时，作家们也创作了许多关于吸血鬼攻击人的恐怖故事。

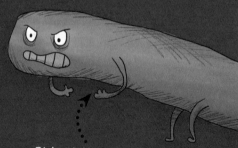

引起结核病的结核分枝杆菌

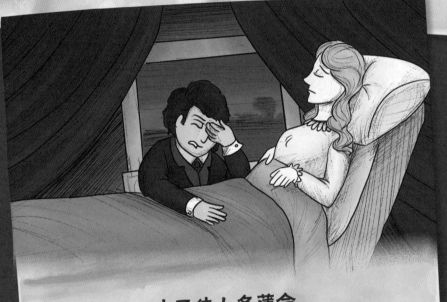

才子佳人多薄命

在19世纪，结核病这种痨病夺去了许多青年诗人和年轻女孩的生命，诗人约翰·济慈就是受害者之一。而在一些人眼里，结核病患者的惨白肤色有一种"令人心悸的美"。于是这种疾病逐渐被赋予了几乎浪漫的色彩。但无论如何，结核病都是让患者饱受折磨的可怕疾病，患者的逝去也让他们的亲友们悲痛欲绝。

昔日的容颜杀手：天花

多亏了疫苗接种的出现，天花现在已经绝迹。而在过去很长一段时间里，天花一直是全世界最可怕的致命疾病之一，患病者即使侥幸活下来，也常会因皮肤留下的皮疹疤痕而毁容。

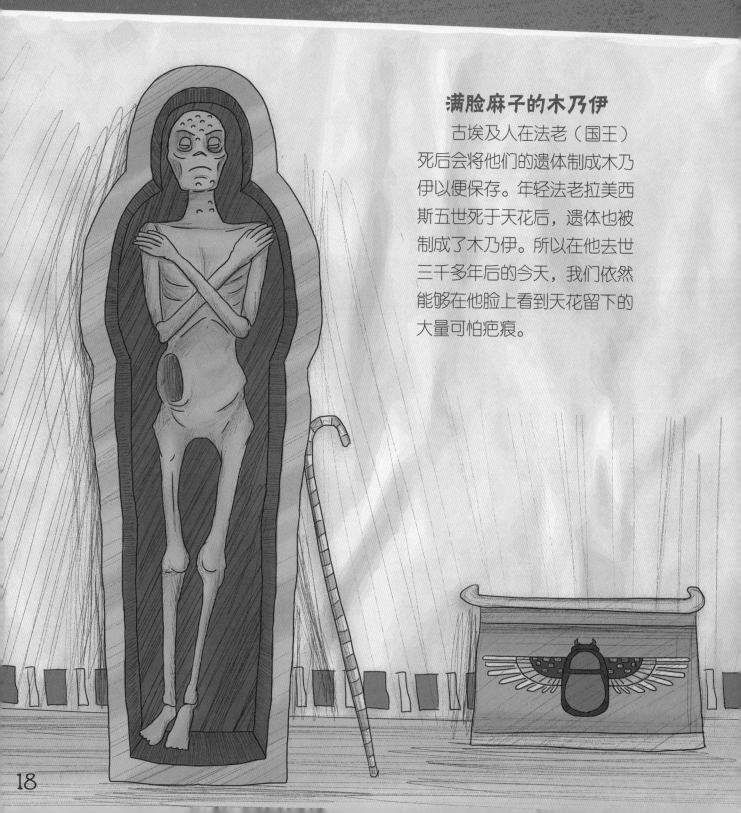

满脸麻子的木乃伊

古埃及人在法老（国王）死后会将他们的遗体制成木乃伊以便保存。年轻法老拉美西斯五世死于天花后，遗体也被制成了木乃伊。所以在他去世三千多年后的今天，我们依然能够在他脸上看到天花留下的大量可怕疤痕。

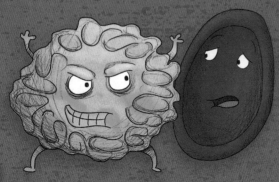

白面女王伊丽莎白

1562年10月，年轻的英格兰女王伊丽莎白一世感染了天花，她曾命悬一线，一周后才脱离危险。虽然她最终挺了过来，但是脸上留下了疤痕，头发也大量脱落。在后来的岁月里，她在脸上涂抹厚厚的白色乳霜来遮盖疤痕，这种白色乳霜是用含铅涂料掺入蛋白调制的。为了掩盖稀疏的头发，她还戴上了假发。

邪恶的天花病毒

天花是由天花病毒引起的。在一万六千年以前，天花病毒从啮齿类动物传到了人身上，然后逐渐变异进化，具备了侵入人体细胞的能力，从而使人患上天花。多亏了疫苗接种的出现，天花病毒已被消灭，只留下了少量样本被安全存储起来。

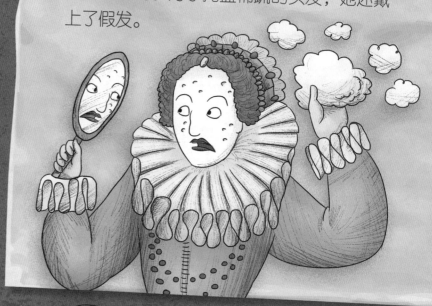

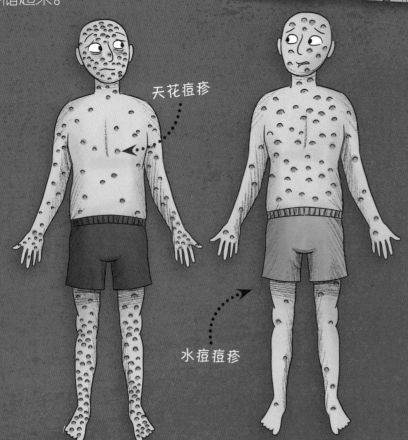

天花痘疹

水痘痘疹

痘疹密布：天花的症状

人感染天花病毒后的头两周不会有什么症状。接下来感染者会觉得自己得了流感，但症状会逐渐减轻。随着病程的发展，感染者面部和前臂会突然出现红色痘疹，之后痘疹会越来越多，蔓延至全身，此时的病情已经非常严重了。天花痘疹看上去像轻微的水痘痘疹，但要比水痘痘疹密集得多。

拿破仑的噩梦：斑疹伤寒

由于疫苗接种的出现，斑疹伤寒跟天花一样，现在也几乎绝迹了。但斑疹伤寒曾经也是和天花一样致命的疾病，会让感染者极度痛苦，且致死率很高。患者一开始的症状类似流感，接下来全身会出现严重的皮疹。

小小微生物击垮数十万大军

法国皇帝拿破仑曾经征服了大半个欧洲。1812年，他又率领军队远征俄国。但在到达莫斯科后，却发现俄军已经撤走，只留下了一座空城，拿破仑只好决定撤军。而在撤军返国途中，法军遭遇了俄国严冬的极寒天气，大批官兵因感染斑疹伤寒而死去，人数远远超过和俄军交战时的战死人数。

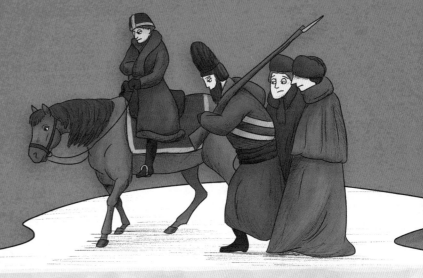

作大恶的小虫子

斑疹伤寒的致病元凶是多种立克次氏体细菌。这些细菌经由动物的粪便或恶心的小虱子、跳蚤感染人类。这些脏污之物会使人全身发痒、抓挠皮肤，也就为这些致病细菌打开了入侵人体的大门。

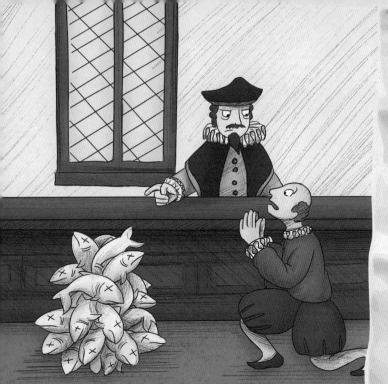

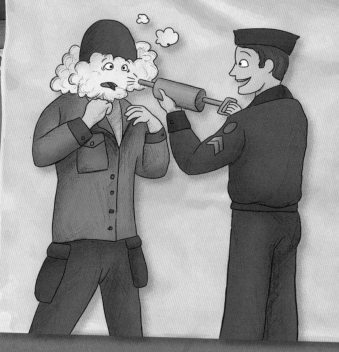

灭虱大作战

第二次世界大战刚刚结束时，斑疹伤寒本来可能在人员密集的兵营和难民聚居点迅速传播。但由于人们在人员密集区域喷洒滴滴涕，得以拯救数百万人的生命。因为这种化学药品滴滴涕（双对氯苯基三氯乙烷）可以杀灭传播斑疹伤寒的虱子。

比坐牢还可怕的"监狱热"

16世纪，许多犯罪嫌疑人还没等到审判，就因斑疹伤寒，也就是"监狱热"，死于狱中。1586年，38名被控偷鱼的渔民被抬上英格兰埃克塞特的法庭受审，其中有一半人因患斑疹伤寒死去，并把斑疹伤寒传染给了许多法庭公务人员。

马铃薯引发的惨祸

在19世纪40年代爱尔兰大饥荒时期，贫苦灾民饱受饥荒折磨，而斑疹伤寒又让他们的处境雪上加霜。当时，爱尔兰普通民众赖以生存的主要作物马铃薯因疫病严重减产，导致大批爱尔兰人挨饿，还有大批居民被迫背井离乡、移民国外。斑疹伤寒从爱尔兰传播到英格兰，因此又得名"爱尔兰热"。

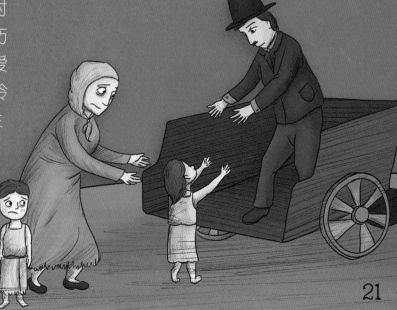

不干不净惹人病：霍乱

霍乱是最可怕的疾病之一，患者会腹泻脱水，造成身体极度虚弱。人们饮用了被霍乱弧菌污染的水后就会感染霍乱，而霍乱弧菌在不洁净的水中可以大量繁殖。

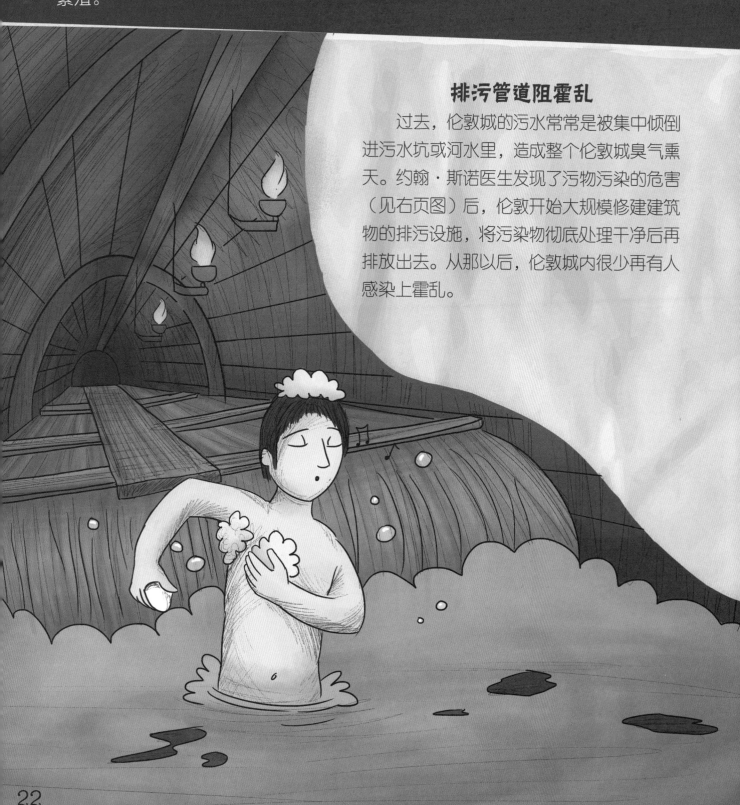

排污管道阻霍乱

过去，伦敦城的污水常常是被集中倾倒进污水坑或河水里，造成整个伦敦城臭气熏天。约翰·斯诺医生发现了污物污染的危害（见右页图）后，伦敦开始大规模修建建筑物的排污设施，将污染物彻底处理干净后再排放出去。从那以后，伦敦城内很少再有人感染上霍乱。

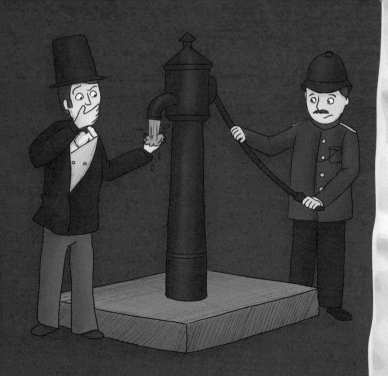

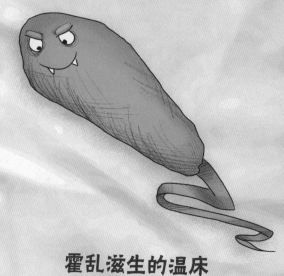

斯诺的重大发现

在1854年伦敦索霍区暴发霍乱疫情之前，没有人知道霍乱的病因。那次霍乱大流行促使约翰·斯诺医生深入调查霍乱的病因。斯诺发现所有病人都饮用了布罗德维克街上一个水泵抽上来的水。原来这个水泵的水源已经被下水道泄漏的污水污染了。

令人胆寒的黄黑旗

19世纪城镇繁荣发展，但城镇清洁用水不足，污水处理系统也不完善，造成了霍乱大范围肆虐。当时，如果一艘船上有人感染了霍乱，该船必须要挂起黄黑相间的旗帜来警告其他船只，且这艘船上的所有人一个月都不许上岸。

霍乱滋生的温床

引起霍乱的霍乱弧菌在被人类粪便污染的食物和水体中会迅速繁殖。人们如果食用了在污染水域里活动的海洋生物，就会感染上霍乱。当人们食用或饮用了含有霍乱病菌的食物或水后，霍乱病菌就会在人的肠道里大量繁殖，引发严重的病症。

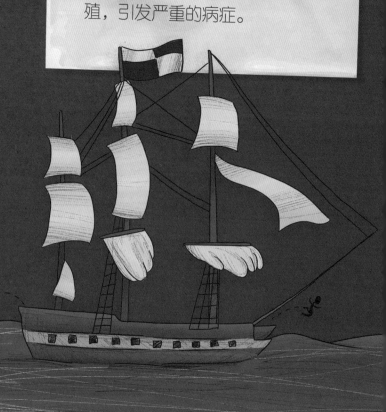

肆虐一时的黄色瘟疫：黄热病

黄热病是一种流行于热带地区的危险疾病，人们染病后会发高烧、呕吐，身体变得虚弱不堪。由于病菌会破坏肝脏细胞，病人有时会出现皮肤变黄的情况。

危险信号：皮肤变黄

大多数情况下，黄热病患者在发热出汗、恶心呕吐几日后病情就会好转。但是会有六分之一的病人出现病毒侵袭肝脏的情况，导致皮肤变黄，腹部疼痛难忍，接着口、眼和肠道也会出血，最后呕出黑血。

黄热病症状

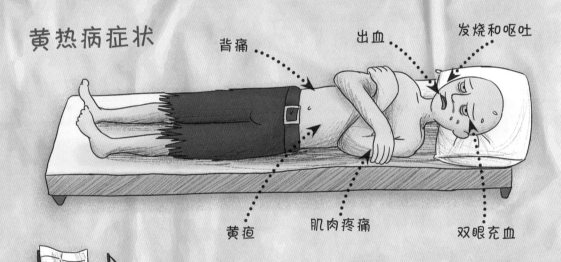

背痛　　出血　　发烧和呕吐

黄疸　　肌肉疼痛　　双眼充血

费城大逃亡

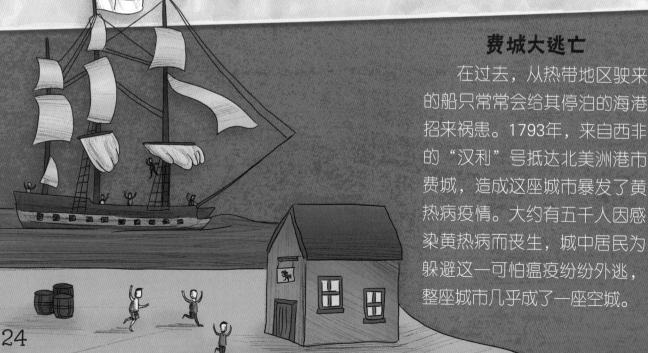

在过去，从热带地区驶来的船只常常会给其停泊的海港招来祸患。1793年，来自西非的"汉利"号抵达北美洲港市费城，造成这座城市暴发了黄热病疫情。大约有五千人因感染黄热病而丧生，城中居民为躲避这一可怕瘟疫纷纷外逃，整座城市几乎成了一座空城。

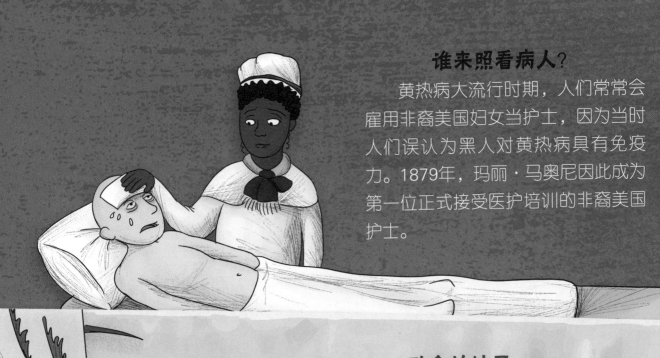

谁来照看病人?

黄热病大流行时期，人们常常会雇用非裔美国妇女当护士，因为当时人们误认为黑人对黄热病具有免疫力。1879年，玛丽·马奥尼因此成为第一位正式接受医护培训的非裔美国护士。

致命的蚊子

黄热病的致病病毒是通过雌性埃及伊蚊叮咬人类传播的。如果这种蚊子叮咬了黄热病感染者后再次叮咬其他人时，会一边吸血一边将唾液和致命的病毒注入被叮咬者的伤口中。寨卡热和登革热也是由埃及伊蚊通过这种方式传播的。

防蚊灭蚊赶瘟疫

人们曾经以为黄热病是人和人之间经由空气传播的。1881年，古巴医生卡洛斯·芬莱向人们证明，恼人的小蚊子才是罪魁祸首。于是人们意识到，一定要避开蚊虫泛滥的地区，晚上睡觉时也应该撑起蚊帐防范蚊虫叮咬。

25

致命的感冒：西班牙流感

大多数情况下，流感只是冬季里一种轻微的疾病，但是有些类型的流感却能使人丧命。1918年至1919年期间，一种被称为"西班牙流感"的恶性流感暴发，夺去了2,000万至4,000万患者的生命，这场流感大流行也成了史上最致命的灾难之一。

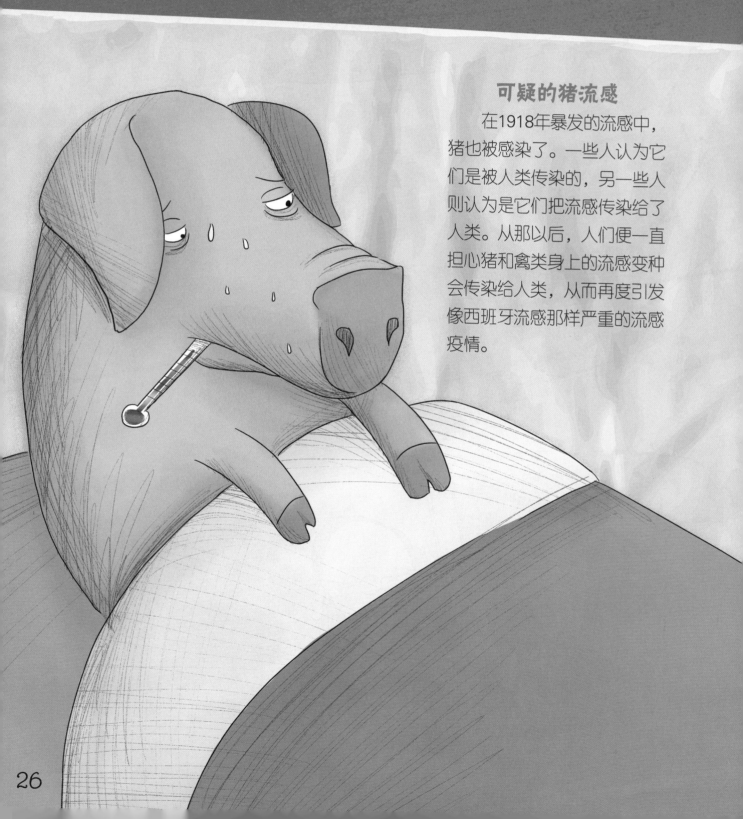

可疑的猪流感

在1918年暴发的流感中，猪也被感染了。一些人认为它们是被人类传染的，另一些人则认为是它们把流感传染给了人类。从那以后，人们便一直担心猪和禽类身上的流感变种会传染给人类，从而再度引发像西班牙流感那样严重的流感疫情。

滋生流感的战壕

第一次世界大战期间，法国泥泞的战壕里挤满数百万士兵。大批生猪也在战壕附近堆积如山，充当士兵的口粮。有人认为，流感病毒在人和猪之间来回传播，从而演变出致命的变种。

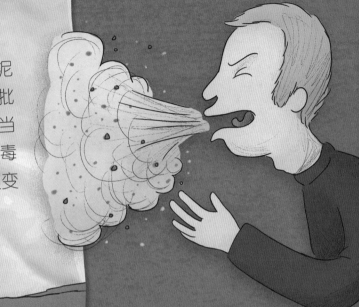

病从天降：飞沫传播

流感的传染性很强，非常容易传播。流感患者只需通过打喷嚏，就能向空中喷出包含大量流感病毒的飞沫，其他人吸入这些飞沫就会染病。在严重流感疫情暴发期间，人们会面戴口罩以避免吸入病菌，但这种预防措施不怎么见效。

死神的第一站：芬斯顿营地

芬斯顿营地听起来像是一个度假胜地，但是，在1918年3月，它无论如何也无法和休闲度假联系起来。当时它是美国堪萨斯州的新兵训练营，据说，可怕的西班牙流感正是从这里开始传播的。

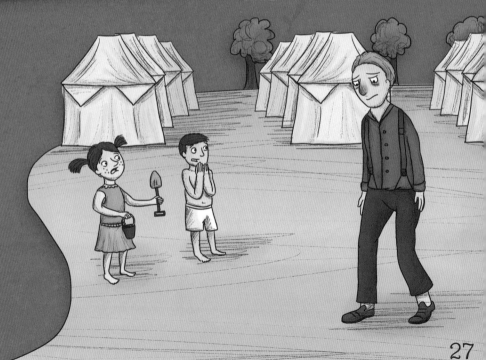

回看历史上的重大疫情

万幸的是，历史上大多数瘟疫流行最后都会平息。新的感染者会逐渐减少，直至再无人感染；已经感染瘟疫的病人也会挺过发病期，恢复健康。但这些可怕的瘟疫还是给人类带来了巨大的苦难。以下记录的是历史上一些曾经肆虐一时的可怕瘟疫之最。

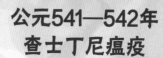

公元541—542年
查士丁尼瘟疫

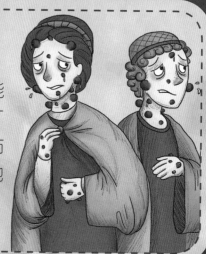

这场瘟疫（很可能是腺鼠疫）从君士坦丁堡（现在的伊斯坦布尔）暴发，之后向其他地区蔓延。

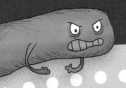

公元前400年

公元600年

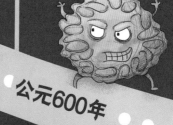

公元前430年
雅典瘟疫

古雅典曾经非常强盛，而一场可怕的瘟疫流行结束了它的黄金时代。专家们认为那次暴发的瘟疫可能是斑疹伤寒，但并不能确定。

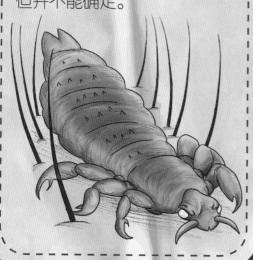

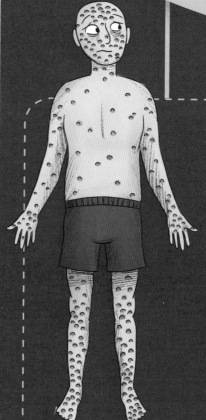

公元165—180年
安东尼瘟疫

公元165年，罗马帝国遭大流行病袭击，造成五百万人死亡，罗马帝国元气大伤。如今，专家们认为这次瘟疫的罪魁祸首可能是天花或麻疹。

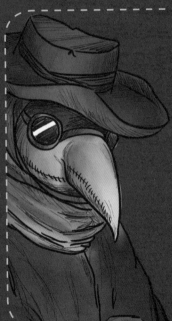

1665—1666年
伦敦大瘟疫

虽然鼠疫多次侵袭人类，但伦敦大瘟疫是欧洲地区最后一次大规模的鼠疫暴发。伦敦的死亡人数达十万人，占当时整个伦敦人口的四分之一。

1918—1919年 西班牙流感

第一次世界大战结束不久后，全世界范围内暴发了历史上最严重的一次流感，史称西班牙流感。当时全世界有五分之一的人口感染此流感，死亡人数达到四千万。

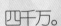

1855年 第三次鼠疫大流行

继查士丁尼瘟疫和黑死病流行之后，又出现了第三次鼠疫大流行。此次鼠疫于1855年开始在中国大规模暴发，之后疫情席卷印度，继而传到美洲。

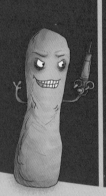

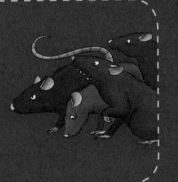

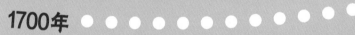

1700年   1900年

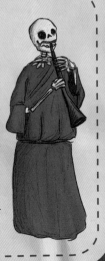

1347—1351年
黑死病流行

黑死病是历史上最可怕的大流行病之一。在短短几年时间里，就有2,500万人——相当于当时欧洲人口的三分之一——被黑死病夺去性命。

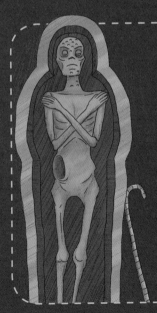

20世纪 天花肆虐

天花在1980年被彻底消灭以前，在20世纪夺去了很多人的生命。天花大概是有史以来最可怕的致命疾病之一。谢天谢地，天花现在再也不能如此逞凶了！

可怕疫病小百科

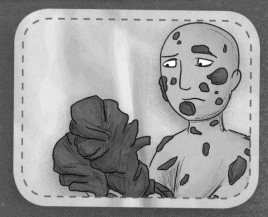

疣状表皮发育不良是一种极罕见的疾病，患者全身会长满大块的疣。

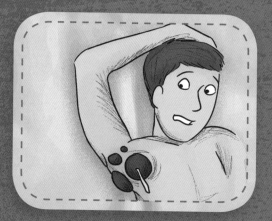

腹股沟淋巴结炎是在腋下、颈部或者腹股沟位置生出的充满脓液的疱，腺鼠疫的发病症状之一就是出现此类疱。

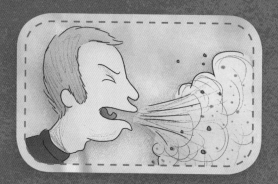

一个喷嚏可以喷出六百万个很小的病毒。

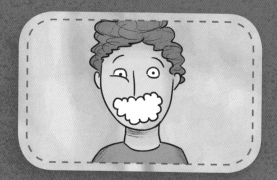

人如果被携带狂犬病病毒的恶犬咬伤，发病时可能会流口水或口吐白沫。

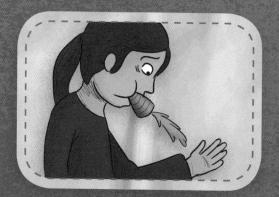

人们呕吐时，即使根本没吃过胡萝卜，也常常会吐出类似胡萝卜的呕吐物。这些其实是脱落的部分胃黏膜。

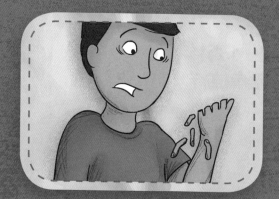

麻风病患者的发病症状非常恐怖，一些患者的手指和脚趾会脱落。麻风病患者曾经被隔离起来，被迫到"麻风病人隔离区"居住。

术语表

白色瘟疫	造成患病者皮肤惨白、无血色的疾病，通常指结核病
大流行病	在全世界范围内暴发的大型传染性疾病
肺鼠疫	与腺鼠疫相关的可怕疾病，不同之处在于病菌会损害肺部，而不是出现腹股沟淋巴结炎
黑死病	14世纪40年代末席卷世界的腺鼠疫可怕大流行病，造成上千万人丧命
琥珀	很久以前树上分泌的树脂凝结而成的固体
痨病	主要侵犯肺部的致命疾病——结核病——的旧称
疟疾	由一种蚊子传播、多发生于热带区域的疾病
疟原虫	一种能使人患疟疾的微生物
微生物	一种极小的、需要用显微镜观察的生物
蚊子	能传播疾病的吸血小昆虫，传播的疾病有疟疾、黄热病等
细菌	一种单细胞微生物
腺鼠疫	由鼠疫杆菌引发的可怕疾病，其特征是感染者常常会出现腹股沟淋巴结炎
疫苗接种	接种失去活性或活性减弱的病菌以刺激免疫系统产生应答，从而预防感染的防疫方法

索引

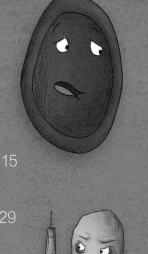

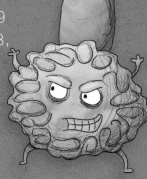

作者简介

约翰·法恩登是位多产的科普图书作家，作品涉及科学、技术和自然领域，包括全球畅销书《放我出去》和《你觉得自己聪明吗？》，并曾五次获得英国皇家学会青少年科学图书奖的提名。

绘者简介

温妮莎·迪安成长于英国布赖顿，从小时候能握住铅笔起就十分热爱绘画。她在19岁生日时收到了一个电子绘画板，便开始尝试电子绘画，从此在这条路上探索不止。

The Grisly History of Medicine
Potions, Poisons and Pills

Written by John Farndon
Illustrated by Venitia Dean

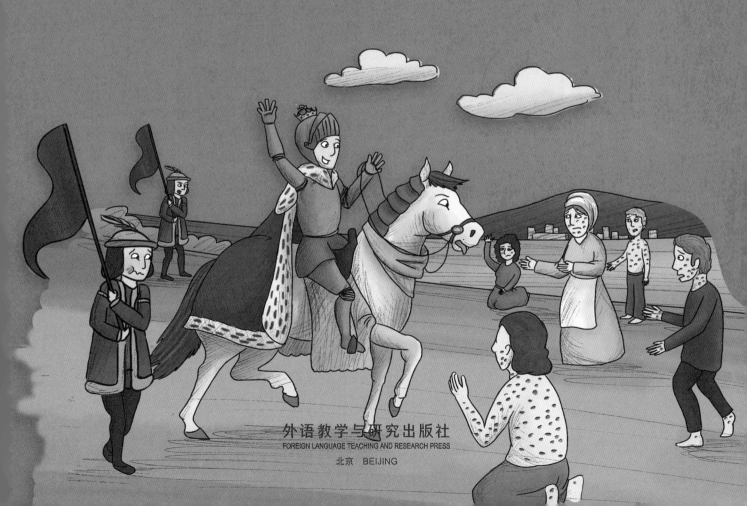

外语教学与研究出版社
FOREIGN LANGUAGE TEACHING AND RESEARCH PRESS
北京 BEIJING

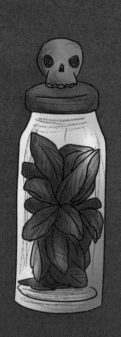
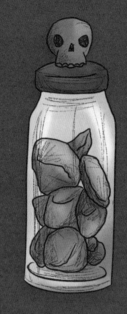
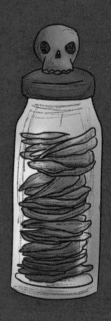

Lots of us take a pill when we have a headache – or worse. But did you know that the art of mixing medicines goes back thousands of years? See inside for the story of daring remedies, yucky cures and truly brilliant ideas for making people better – whatever the problem!

- A venomous snake dissolved in wine cured fatigue and hair loss
- Snail slime was used for burns and roast kittens for jaundice
- Chewing willow bark eased pain and malaria
  ...

Discover how herbal medicine was practised centuries ago, deadly syphilis was cured with Paul Ehrlich's 'magic bullet', and cockroaches, catfish and frogs make their own antibiotics. There are many natural (and other) remedies out there and scientists never stop looking!

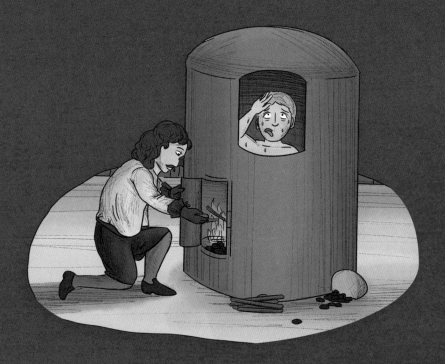

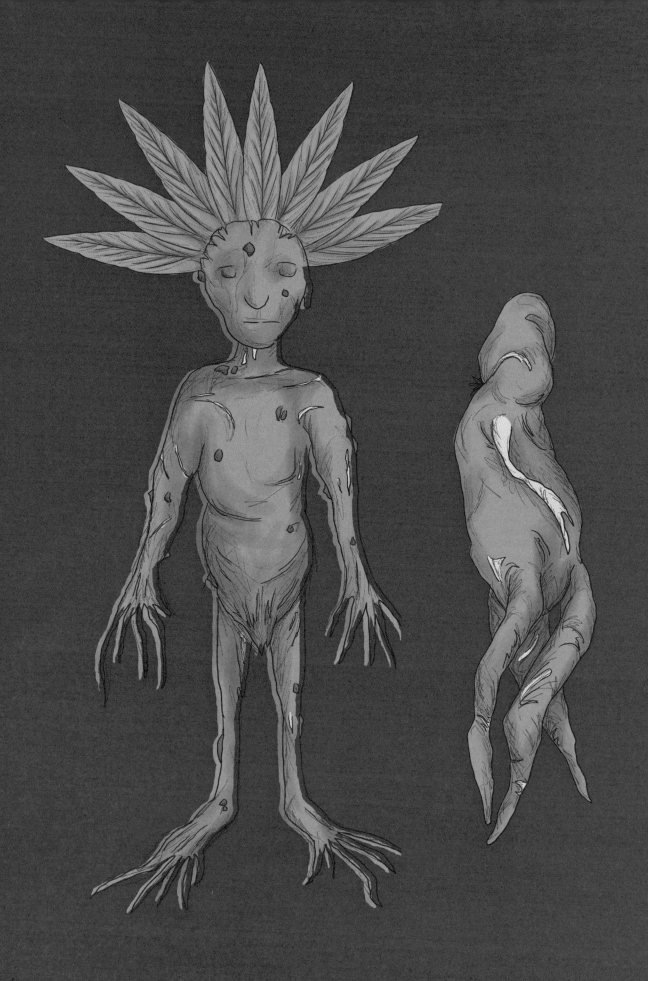

4

Contents

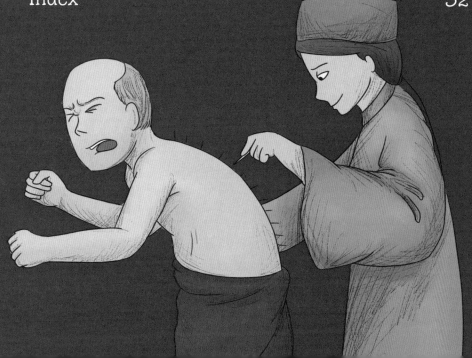

INTRODUCTION

When someone gets sick, they need the right medicine to help them get better. But just what is the right medicine? That's a problem that has been plaguing doctors since ancient times. In this book, we explore some of the great ideas they have come up with, and some of the very bad...

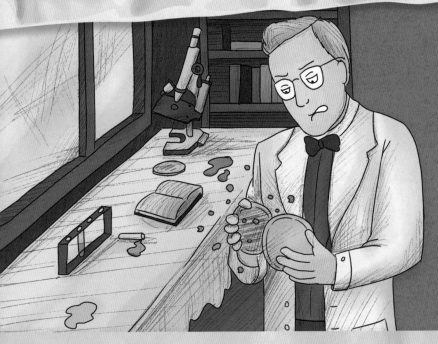

Germ killers

Some medicines are designed to help people get better by fighting infections. Antibiotics, for instance, are medicines that kill or attack the germs that make people ill. Antibiotics only work against bacteria. To fight viruses, you need special antiviral drugs.

Correcting mistakes

Sometimes the body makes too much or too little of certain chemicals. Some medicines are designed to replace missing chemicals, or block their production when the body is making too much. Diabetics, for instance, are given insulin (which used to be taken from the pancreases of pigs) to replace the insulin their bodies are unable to make.

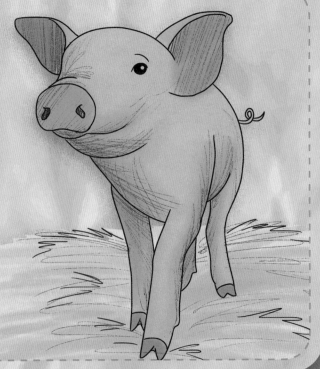

Soothing the symptoms

Some medicines are not meant to cure people; they are just designed to make them feel better by relieving symptoms. Pain relievers, for instance, can make headaches or sore throats less painful. Creams can make skin less itchy.

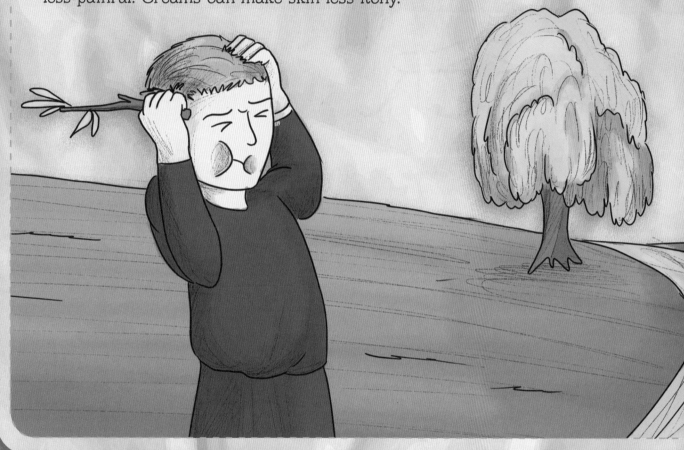

Medical business

It is said that Americans use as much medicine as all the rest of the world put together. Every year, they buy and use a third of a trillion dollars' worth of medicines! In other words, every single American uses a thousand dollars' worth of drugs every year. So they must be very well, or very sick...

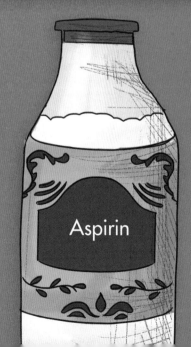

Aspirin

ANCIENT MEDICINE

Many herbs and natural materials have healing properties. But people learnt long ago that these natural medicines can often be made more effective by preparing them or mixing them in certain ways. This ancient art of pharmacy dates back to Ancient Egypt and beyond.

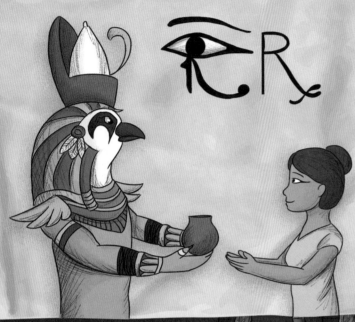

The father of pharmacy

The Ancient Egyptians believed pharmacy began with the god Horus. Horus lost his eye in an epic battle, but it was healed by the god Thoth. Pharmacists today write the sign 'Rx' on prescriptions for medicine. Some believe they are writing the ancient sign for the eye of Horus. Others think that 'Rx' is just medieval shorthand for the Latin for 'recipe'.

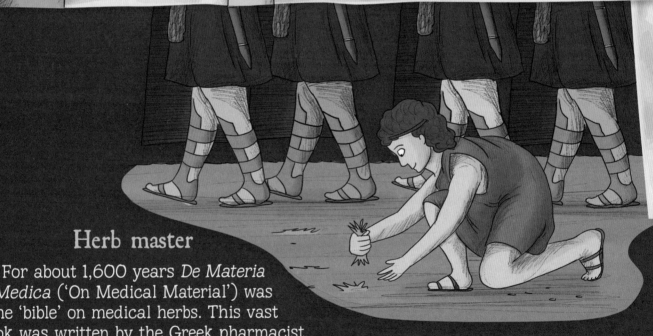

Herb master

For about 1,600 years *De Materia Medica* ('On Medical Material') was the 'bible' on medical herbs. This vast book was written by the Greek pharmacist Dioscorides in the 1st century AD. It describes nearly 600 herbal medicines, many discovered by Dioscorides himself as he followed Roman armies round Europe.

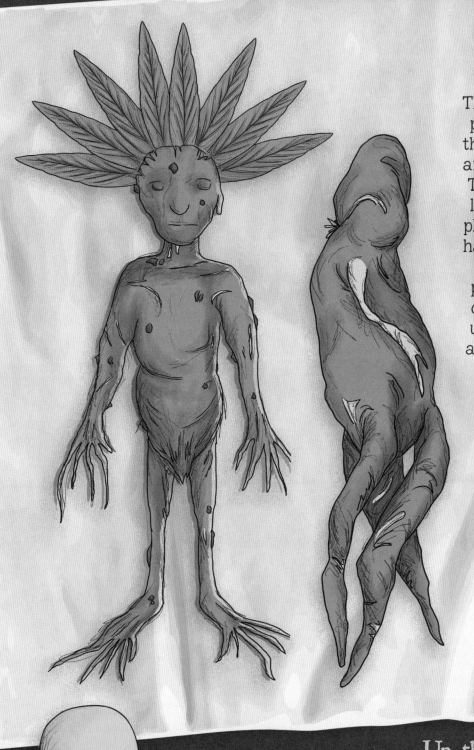

Screaming root

The root of the mandrake plant is a powerful drug that causes hallucinations and sends people to sleep. The roots can be shaped like a little man and the plant was long thought to have magic powers. Some said it screamed when pulled from the ground, cursing the person who uprooted it, so they tied a poor dog to it to pull it up instead.

Up the back

We take most drugs through our mouths, but long ago some doctors had the idea of putting them into the body from the other end. Basically, they stuck a tube called a 'clyster pipe' into the patient's bottom. Then they attached a tube to squirt the medicine in. Nowadays, doctors still use this method, only they call it an 'enema'.

9

CHINESE ROOTS

The Chinese have an ancient tradition of looking for cures in nature. But they don't just use herbs for medicine – they have used all kinds of other strange things, too, from scorpion stings to centipedes.

Live forever!

For many centuries, Chinese chemists searched for a pill that would make people live forever. One story tells that a man called Wei Bo-yang did succeed in making an 'immortality' pill. The story also says that the legendary Yellow Emperor, Huangdi, found this pill and so lived on forever.

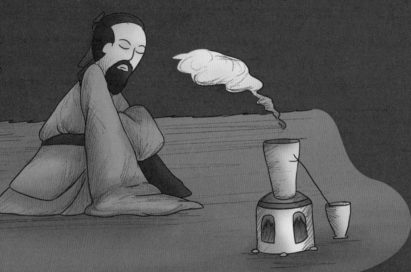

The point of medicine

Acupuncture involves sticking sharp needles into the skin. Ouch! The needles are meant to activate healing pathways or 'meridians' in the body. Acupuncture has been practised in China for more than 2,000 years, and it may have been known in Europe long ago, too. 'Ötzi', a man from about 5,000 years ago, found frozen in mountain ice, has tattoos that seem to mark acupuncture meridians.

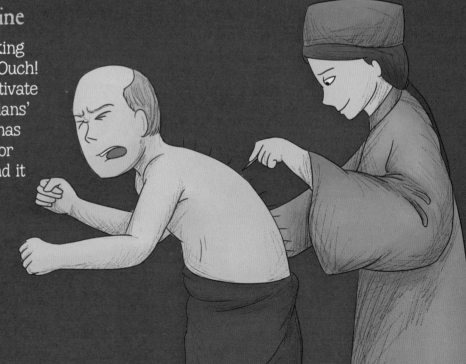

This medicine stings!

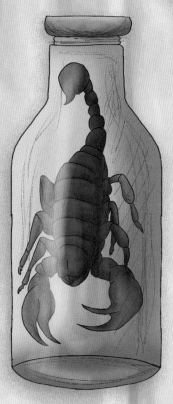

Most of us would steer well clear of scorpions. The sting in their tail is always painful, and can be deadly. Yet the Chinese have long believed that pickled scorpions, or *quan xie*, can cure fits, headaches and swelling. But maybe patients just said 'I'm better!' as soon as they saw the medicine they were being given!

Snake wine

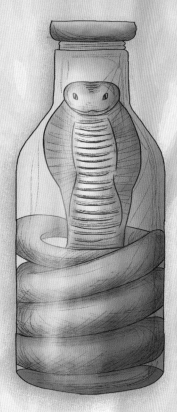

If you're feeling a little tired, or you're losing your hair, what you need is snake wine, according to ancient Chinese medicine. Snake wine is made by drowning a venomous snake in rice wine! It was first used nearly 2,800 years ago.

Killing sea horses

Sea horses are beautiful marine creatures that are in danger of extinction. Yet those who believe in traditional Chinese medicine buy 25 million of them every year. They are convinced dried sea horses can cure kidney complaints, wheezing, tummy aches and much more.

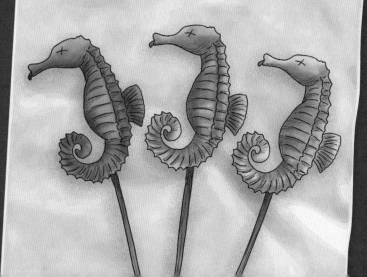

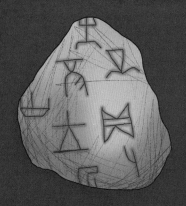

Dragon bones

The fossilised bones of long-dead creatures are often called 'dragon bones' in China. Ground to a powder, they are used in Chinese medicine to cure heart problems, stress and fever. In the ancient past, dragon bones, or 'oracle bones', were also scratched with questions that people wanted to ask the gods.

IT'S CHEMISTRY

Most modern medicines are made from chemicals rather than herbs, and we owe this to the scientists of Ancient Islam. It all started with the brilliant Jābir ibn Hayyān, also known as Geber, who may have lived in Kūfah (in modern Iraq) 1,300 years ago.

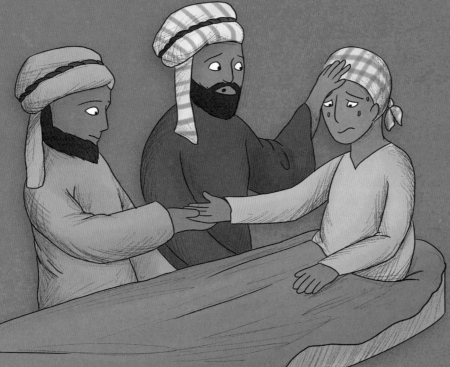

Bedside manner

To get just the right mix of chemicals to make the medicine, the Islamic physicians believed they needed to spend time with each patient and find out all they could about their symptoms and character.

Take your poison

It is said that Jābir knew all there was to know at that time about the chemistry of poisons. In his famous *Book of Poisons*, he described hundreds of toxic substances, and how they react in the body. He also described 'antidotes' – substances that work against the effects of poison – and gave practical demonstrations of them in action.

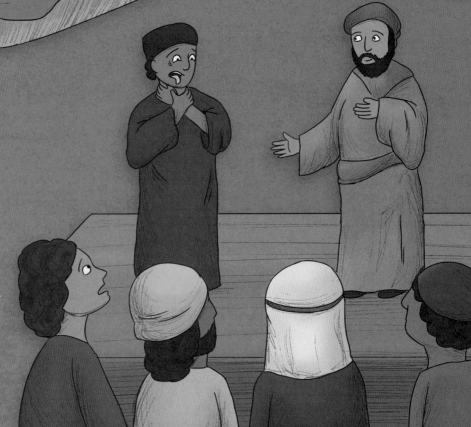

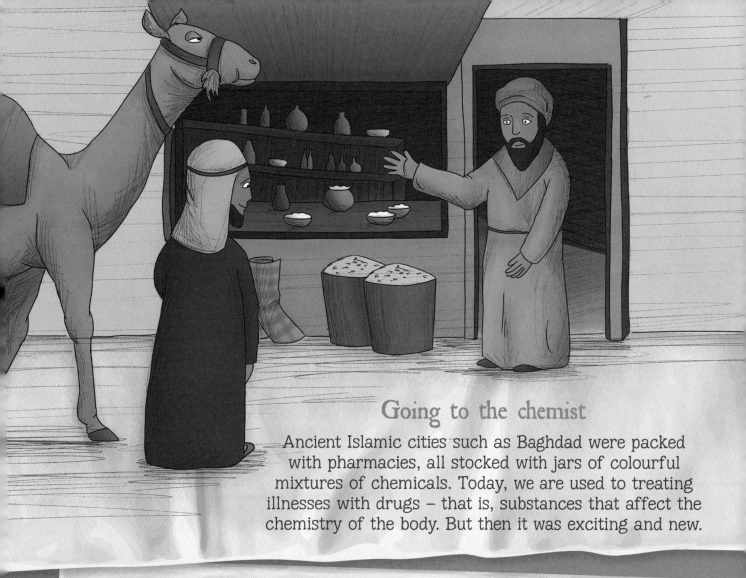

Going to the chemist

Ancient Islamic cities such as Baghdad were packed with pharmacies, all stocked with jars of colourful mixtures of chemicals. Today, we are used to treating illnesses with drugs – that is, substances that affect the chemistry of the body. But then it was exciting and new.

Poison, madam?

Many medicines included deadly poisons, such as henbane, hemlock and black nightshade. Ancient chemists weren't trying to kill the sick. In fact, they'd made a crucial discovery: what matters with giving medicines is the dose. In small doses, some poisons are powerful drugs for relieving pain or sending you to sleep. But they didn't always get the dose right. Bye bye!

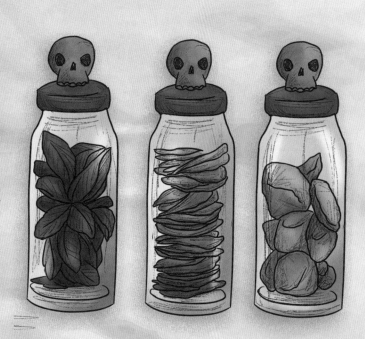

PLUCKED OWLS AND ROAST KITTENS

In the Middle Ages, only the very, very rich had a doctor. If you were ill, you went to the apothecary. Apothecaries were like today's pharmacists, but they not only told you what was wrong with you – they prepared their own medicines.

Secret recipes

Apothecaries' shops were packed with all kinds of mysterious jars and weird ingredients. Apothecaries liked to keep recipes secret, so some ingredients may have been deliberately misleading... All the same, you might find plucked and boiled owls (for gout), hedgehog grease (for a throat infection), snail slime (for burns) and roast kittens (for jaundice).

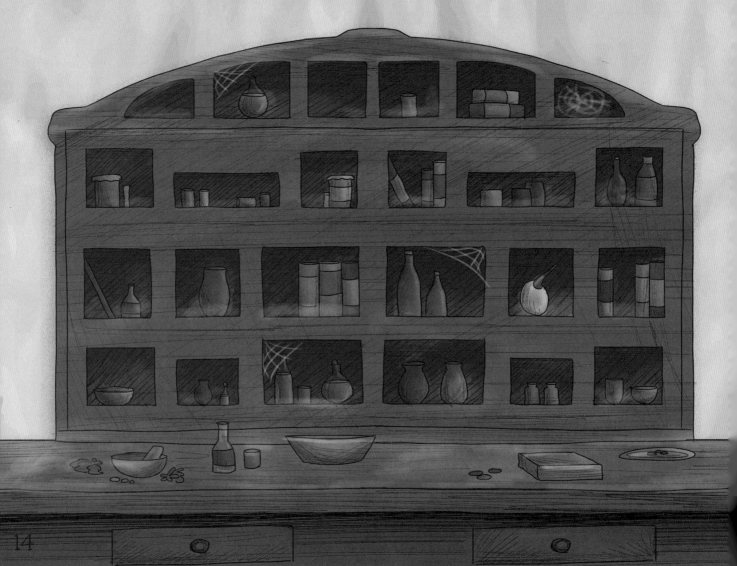

Medical mix

To make a medicine, the apothecary weighed out his chosen ingredients in scales. He ground dry ingredients to a powder in a sturdy bowl called a 'mortar', with a stick called a 'pestle'. He purified and concentrated liquids in a kind of kettle known as an 'alembic'.

Ear this

It seemed everything that falls off your body could be mixed into medicine, too – hair, fingernails, saliva (for skin irritations), old bits of skin... If you suffered from bad headaches, some apothecaries would recommend a nice mix of earwax and mud, usually applied as a balm.

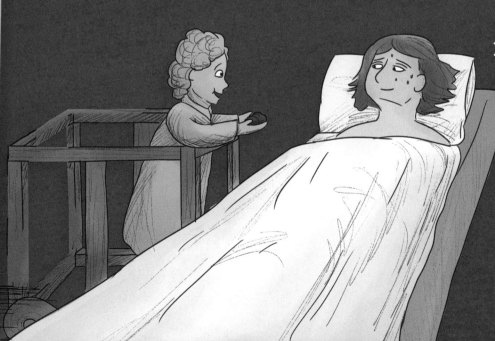

Poo or pee?

Some apothecaries' cures were awful. If you had a sore throat, some would mix you a nice spoonful of dog or baby poo with a dollop of honey. Mind you, if you suffered back pain, they might mix a cup of pee with ox bile, herbs and suet. And for a fever, you might have to sip pig pee...

15

GREEN MEDICINE

The chemicals and exotic ingredients used by apothecaries were hard to come by or very expensive. So for centuries, most people relied on herbs for their medicine. These could be picked from the wild or grown in 'physic' gardens.

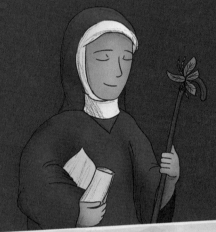

Hildegard's herbs

One of the most famous books on herbal medicine was written by a 12th-century German nun, Hildegard of Bingen, who also happened to be one of the first known musical composers. Hildegard believed in 'green power', using plants and herbs to cure a number of illnesses. Her books are still referred to today.

Garden of medicine

Monasteries set up physic gardens for growing herbs to treat the sick, as well as provide food flavouring and dyes. There were different areas for plants to treat coughs and colds, liver and bladder complaints, digestion, headaches, anxiety and depression, and others.

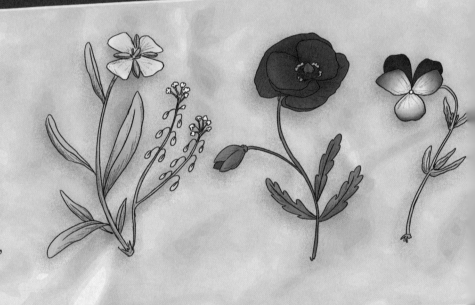

Powerful burdock

Nicholas Culpeper wrote one of the best books on herbal medicine in 1653. But even Culpeper had some odd ideas. He thought that the herb burdock would prevent farting and rabies, and also cure snake bites. He even thought that if women wore it on their heads it would stop their wombs collapsing...

Lookalikes

It was hard to know what substances would heal what ailments. Many people believed in the 'doctrine of signatures'. This was the idea that plants and foods would work as treatments for parts of the body that they look like. So since a sliced mushroom looks like an ear, it must be good for hearing.

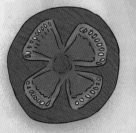
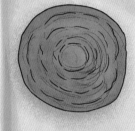
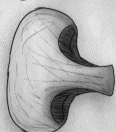
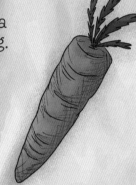

Slice of tomato –
for the heart

Slice of carrot –
for eyes

Slice of mushroom –
for hearing

Whole carrot –
for the nose

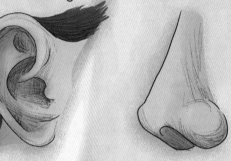

Wise woman

In many country villages, if someone was ill, they went to see the witch, who knew all about herbs. For some people, a witch was just a wise old woman who knew how to heal the sick. But other people were afraid of witches' skill and believed they served the devil.

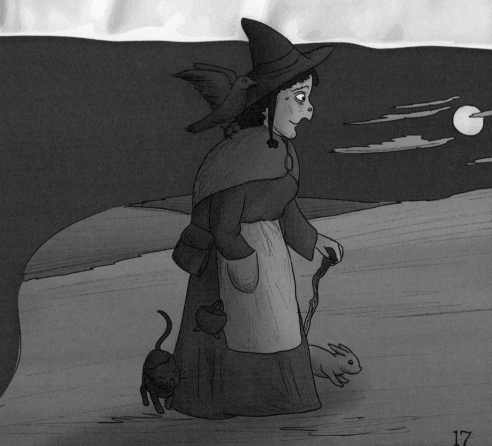

WILLOW POWER

If someone has a bad headache or another pain, it's easy for them to take aspirin or other painkillers. But it wasn't always that way...

Barking mad

Aspirin is made from the chemical salicylic acid. A form of salicylic acid occurs naturally in the bark of willow trees, myrtle and meadowsweet plants. But getting it out of a tree is a real headache...

Taming the snake

Ague (probably malaria) was so nasty that people pictured it as a snake gripping you! Chewing on cinchona bark helped, but this wasn't easy to get in England. Then in 1758, Oxfordshire vicar Edward Stone noticed that willow bark tasted a bit like cinchona bark. He tried it on a few ague victims and they felt better at once.

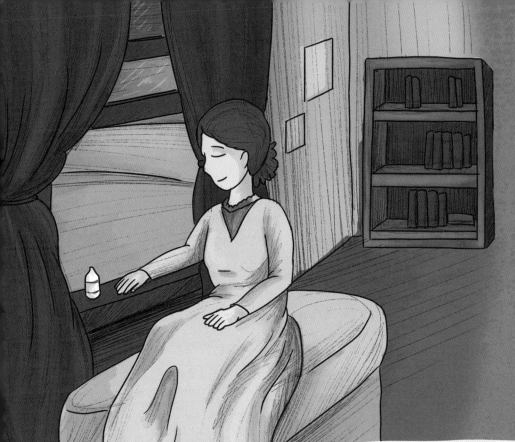

Drugged up

In the 1800s, if someone was in pain, doctors would prescribe a glass of laudanum. This certainly eased the pain, but it was a strong, addictive drug related to heroin. So many who took it became desperate drug addicts, including many women who took it simply to ease period pains.

Aspirin

The pain-relieving ingredient in willow bark is a chemical called salicylic acid. But it attacks the stomach. In the 1890s, Bayer company scientists made the wonder drug aspirin by modifying salicylic acid to make it less damaging. No pain, big gain.

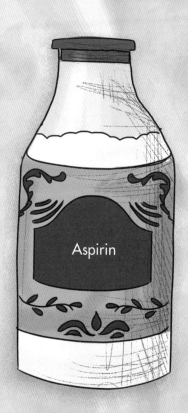

Aspirin

FINDING A MAGIC BULLET

Syphilis is a terrible disease that once ravaged Europe. There seemed to be no cure – until a German physician found a chemical that killed the germs but left the patient unharmed. For him, it was like the mythical 'magic bullet' that kills only the baddie.

We've won!

French king Charles VIII was rather pleased when he marched his conquering army into Naples in Italy in 1495. But his soldiers caught the horrific disease syphilis in the city and spread it across Europe.

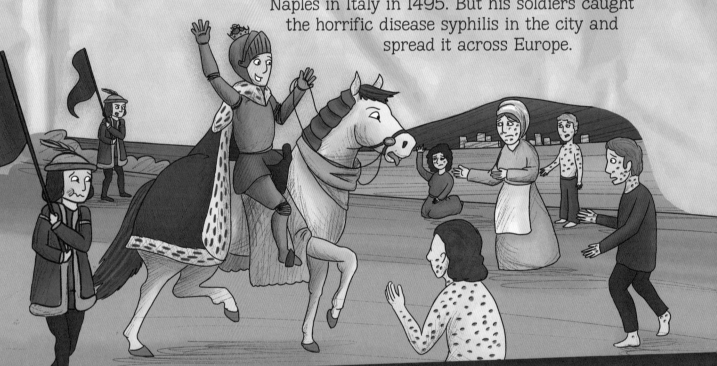

Nose job

Syphilis didn't often kill people straight off, but its effects were really horrible. It made the body burst out with boils so foul that syphilis came to be known as the Great Pox. And it rotted away the nose, so that many syphilis victims had to have artificial noses. It could make the sufferers mad, too.

Fume it out

People were so desperate to be cured of syphilis that they tried almost everything. The metal mercury was thought to help, and one idea was to sit in a box filled with mercury vapour. But mercury is poisonous, and its effects were painful, unpleasant and even fatal.

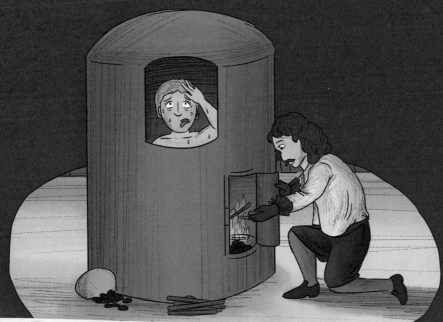

The deaf composer

The brilliant composer Ludwig van Beethoven (1770–1827) went deaf as he got older, so it became very hard for him to write music. People have wondered if his deafness was caused by syphilis. Other possible syphilis victims from history include Henry VIII, Adolf Hitler and the Russian writer Leo Tolstoy.

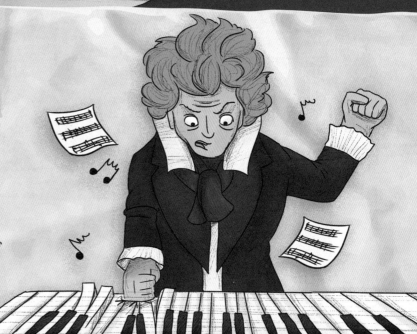

On target

The German scientist Paul Ehrlich (1854–1915) believed that if bacteria could be stained colours by certain dyes, then they might also be killed by them, as if by 'magic bullets'. He and his colleagues tried hundreds of stains and then found one that worked against syphilis germs. They used it to make the drug Salvarsan, the first effective treatment of the disease.

MOULDY NOT DEADLY

Food that's gone mouldy looks pretty yucky, and you wouldn't want to eat it. But it was in mould that Scottish scientist Alexander Fleming discovered the amazing medicine penicillin.

Nasty Staphy

The bacterium *Staphylococcus aureus* is among the world's most common germs. One in five people around the world may carry it on their skin and up their nose. It doesn't always make people ill, but when it does, it's nasty. Meningitis, pneumonia, osteomyelitis (a bone disease), flu, boils and much more are all due to *S. aureus*!

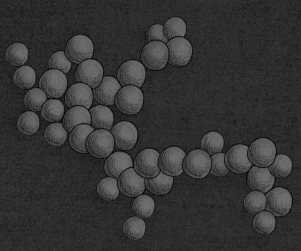

Mould mayhem

In 1928, Fleming went away on holiday while studying *S. aureus* germs in dishes in his laboratory. When he came back, some dishes had gone mouldy. Then he spotted that germs had died where the mould had grown – and realised the mould contained a natural germ-killing substance, which he dubbed 'penicillin'.

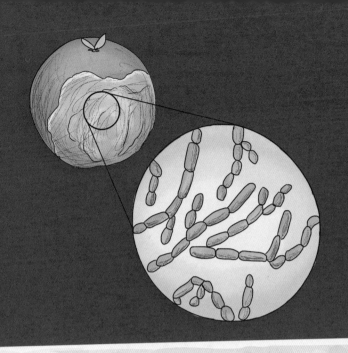

What is penicillin?

The mould *Penicillium notatum*, in which Fleming found penicillin, belongs to a group of fungi. Like all moulds, it grows in tiny threads called 'hyphae' and spreads through the air in minute spores (like seeds). The green fur on a mouldy orange is *P. digitatum*. The blue veins in blue cheese are *P. roqueforti*.

Invasion force

Scientists Howard Florey and Ernst Chain turned Fleming's penicillin into a medicine that would save thousands of lives. They found how to make it in large quantities, so it could be used to treat infected wounds. This saved the lives of countless soldiers injured in the D-Day landings of 1944 in World War II.

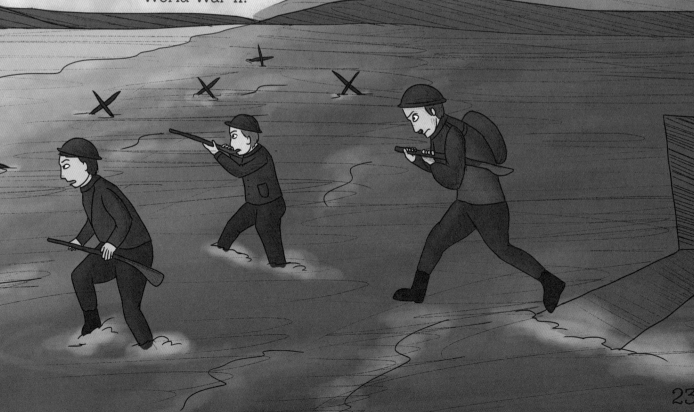

NATURAL KILLERS

Since Fleming discovered penicillin, scientists have discovered thousands of 'antibiotics' – drugs that attack bacteria. Most antibiotics are now entirely man-made. But many were often originally found, like penicillin, in natural sources. The antibiotics tetracycline and streptomycin both came from bacteria. And the natural world is full of antibiotic substances that may inspire new drugs. Here are some of the weirdest places that scientists are looking...

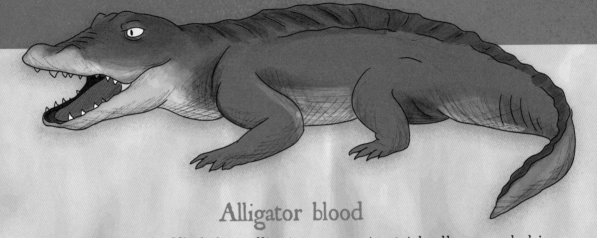

Alligator blood

Scientists were baffled that alligators seem to get badly wounded in fights with other alligators, yet their wounds didn't become infected. When they investigated, they found alligator blood contains natural antibiotics effective against a wide range of infections.

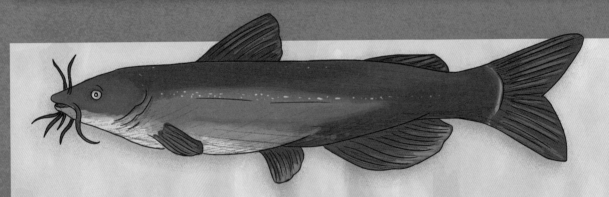

Catfish slime

Catfish seem to survive injuries without getting infected, and scientists found out why. Their bodies are covered in a kind of slime rich in antibiotics that seem to be good at killing off germs such as *Klebsiella pneumoniae*, which attacks the lungs, and *E. coli*.

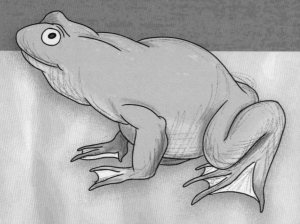

Frog skin

Frogs can survive in water that would kill a lot of creatures. Scientists now know one reason why: their skins are covered in 100 bacteria-killing substances. Yet most are also dangerous to humans, so scientists must find a way to apply their germ-killing powers without hurting us!

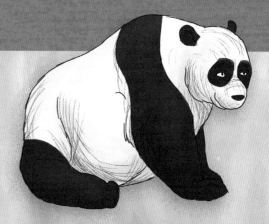

Panda blood

One of the most powerful of all antibiotics, cathelicidin-AM, occurs in panda blood. It kills off germs in a fraction of the time it takes most other antibiotics. But pandas are very rare, so scientists make synthetic panda blood to conduct experiments with cathelicidin-AM.

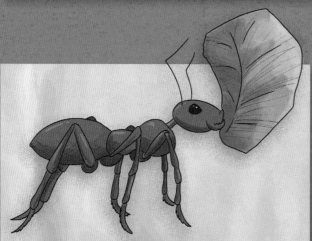

Leafcutter ants

Leafcutter ants are known for their supersize strength in carrying leaves, but they also have superpowers against germs. Scientists have found that their bodies deploy multiple chemicals to fight bacteria and fungi, just as doctors use multi-drug approaches to treat difficult infections.

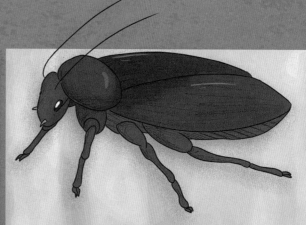

Cockroach brains

Crushed cockroach brains contain nine different kinds of antibiotics. Scientists are trying to find out if some may be used to treat *E. coli* infections or even MRSA: infection by the *S. aureus* 'superbug' bacterium that has become resistant to other antibiotics.

SUGAR IN THE BLOOD

A person who has diabetes can't keep down the sugar levels in their blood. The problem lies with the body chemical insulin, which should control sugar levels, but doesn't. That's why diabetics – people with diabetes – must receive regular injections of insulin.

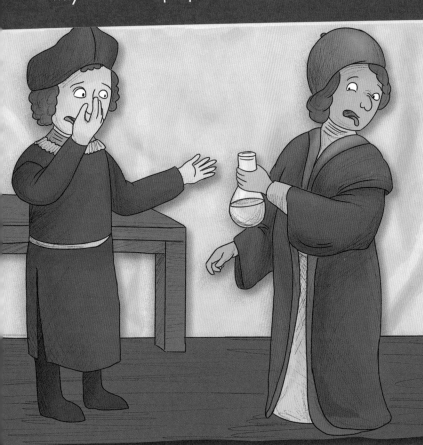

Sweet pees

In the Middle Ages, many doctors knew just how to diagnose diabetes. They tasted the patient's pee. If it tasted sweet, the patient had diabetes. But they hadn't much idea how to treat the disease. Some suggested drinking wine, some eating a lot of sour food and others riding horses!

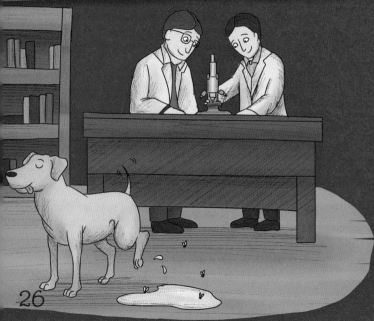

Finding insulin

In 1889, German scientists Oscar Minkowski and Joseph von Mering removed a dog's pancreas for their studies of digestion. Later they saw flies feeding on the dog's pee, found it was sweet and realised that it is the pancreas that controls sugar levels. In 1921, Canadian Frederick Banting and American Charles H. Best discovered that it does this by making insulin.

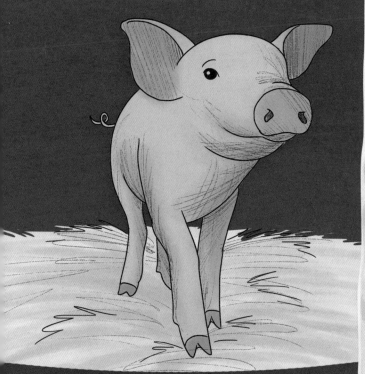

Bacteria factory

In the 1970s, scientists found how to use bacteria as factories for making human insulin. They inserted the gene for human insulin into *E. coli* bacteria, then put them in a huge vat to multiply. As they multiplied, the bacteria followed their new genes' instructions and made lots of human insulin. This is now the main source of insulin for diabetics.

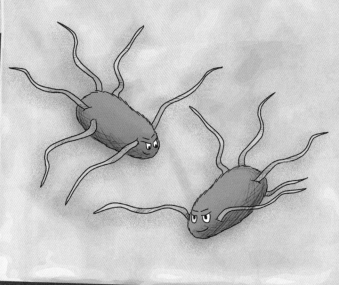

Sweet pigs

The discovery of insulin was a major breakthrough for the treatment of diabetes. Insulin could be extracted from the pancreases of pigs and cows killed for meat. Then it was refined and given to diabetics in injections that kept their condition under control.

Out of the box

Pandora was the mythical girl who was so curious that she opened a box and let out things that would hurt mankind, such as war and disease. Some scientists were worried that genetically modified (GM) bacteria for making insulin might escape and spread – just like 'opening Pandora's box'. At a conference in 1975, they agreed they should never work with disease-causing bacteria, and always work in a completely secure room.

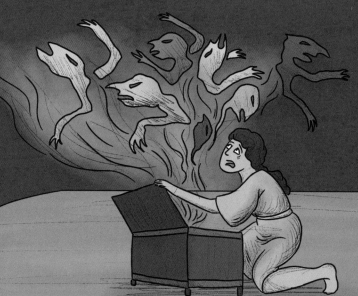

27

MEDICINE THROUGH TIME

Medicines have come a long way, from the simple herbs used in ancient times to the mass-produced chemical drugs of today. Here are some milestones in their development.

About 1520 Dose

German-Swiss scholar Paracelsus was a bit of a weirdo who liked creating mysteries, but it was he who established that medicines (and poisons) must be administered in the right doses to have the right effects.

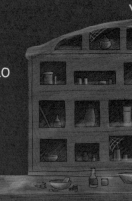

1000 BC

1000

About 2800 BC Divine farmer-cy

Shennong, also known as the Divine Farmer, was a mythical ruler of China who tested the medical effects of hundreds of herbs, and laid the foundations of Chinese traditional medicine still followed today.

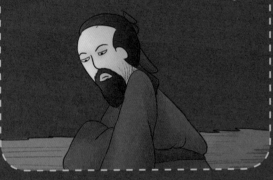

About 800 AD Poison king

Persian chemist Jābir ibn Hayyān wrote one of the first great books on the chemistry of medicines in his *Book of Poisons*.

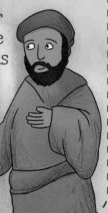

About 60 AD Medical material

The Greek physician Dioscorides wrote a five-volume guide to the medical effects of herbs and other substances called *De Materia Medica* ('On Medical Material').

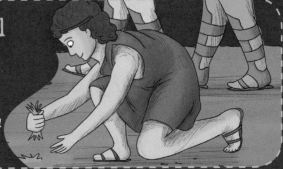

1899 Counter pain

The Bayer chemical company introduced aspirin, one of the first widely sold everyday painkilling medicines.

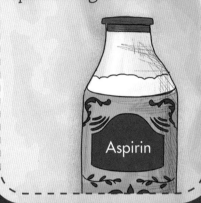

Aspirin

1921 Sweet discovery

Frederick Banting, Charles Best and John Macleod discovered insulin – the chemical produced by the pancreas that controls levels of sugar in the blood – and that diabetes could be treated with injections of artificial insulin.

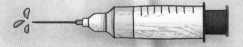

1800   2000

1928 Medicine from mould

Scottish doctor Alexander Fleming discovered penicillin, one of the first known natural bacteria killers or antibiotics, in mould.

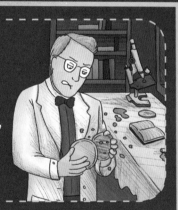

1910 Magic bullet

Salvarsan was the first 'magic bullet' drug, designed to target the bacteria that cause disease. It was the first effective treatment for syphilis.

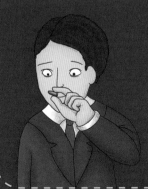

1948 Sore losers

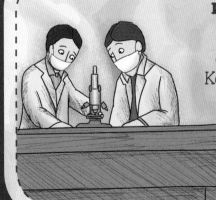

Corticosteroid drugs, discovered by Edward Kendall and Philip Hench, reduce inflammation, which is a key symptom of ailments such as rheumatism.

THE RIGHT PRESCRIPTION

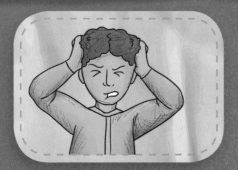

For headaches and low spirits, medieval herbalists gave concoctions including the herbs betony and vervain. Scientists have now discovered that both of these contain chemicals good for treating migraines and depression.

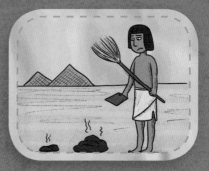

According to one ancient papyrus, the Ancient Egyptians used donkey, dog, gazelle and fly poo as medicines, taken through the mouth.

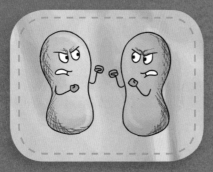

Since the discovery of antibiotics, more and more bacteria have developed resistance to them, primarily through overuse.

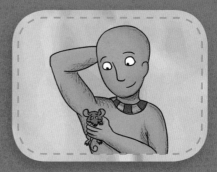

The Ancient Egyptians used lizard blood, dead mice, mud and mouldy bread as ointments for sores.

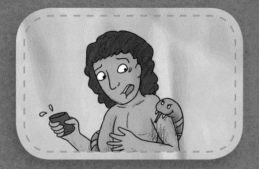

According to legend, the Ancient Greek king Mithridates developed an antidote to all poisons. The Romans turned it into 'theriac', a drug that would cure all ailments. It didn't work, but people continued using it until the late 1800s.

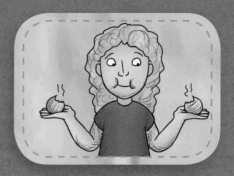

Recently, scientists tested a medieval eye cure made from onions, garlic, wine and bull's gall bladder juice. It looked yucky but had amazing antibacterial properties.

GLOSSARY

Acupuncture	An ancient Chinese treatment involving inserting needles into the body
Alembic	A kind of kettle with a long spout, used by apothecaries for purifying liquids
Antibiotic	A drug that attacks bacteria
Apothecary	Someone who mixed and sold medicines in the past
Bacterium	(plural: bacteria) A microbe made from just one cell
Clyster pipe	A pipe for injecting fluids and gases up a patient's bottom for medical purposes
Doctrine of signatures	The idea that treatments for different parts of the body can be identified by similar shapes in nature
Insulin	The body chemical that regulates levels of sugar in the blood
Laudanum	An addictive painkilling drink made by mixing the drug opium in alcohol
Mortar	A bowl used by apothecaries for grinding and mixing medicines
Penicillin	A substance in the *Penicillium* mould that kills bacteria
Pestle	A stick used by apothecaries for grinding medicine to a powder in a mortar
Salicylic acid	A substance found in meadowsweet and the bark of willow trees, used to reduce inflammation, and also to make aspirin

Index

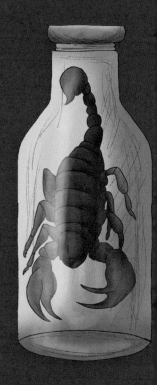

The Author

John Farndon is the author of many books on science, technology and nature, including the international best-sellers *Do Not Open* and *Do You Think You're Clever?* He has been shortlisted five times for the Royal Society's Young People's Book Prize.

The Illustrator

Venitia Dean grew up in Brighton, UK. She has loved drawing ever since she could hold a pencil. After receiving a digital drawing tablet for her 19th birthday she transferred to working digitally. She hasn't looked back since!

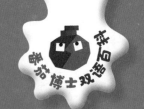

怪诞**医学史**

良药还是毒药?

约翰·法恩登〔英〕 著

温妮莎·迪安〔英〕 绘

向含玥 译

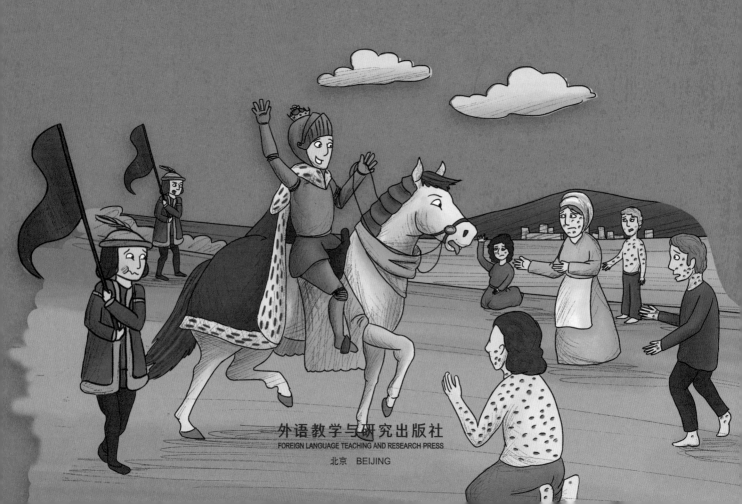

外语教学与研究出版社
FOREIGN LANGUAGE TEACHING AND RESEARCH PRESS
北京 BEIJING

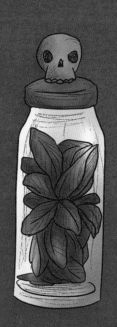
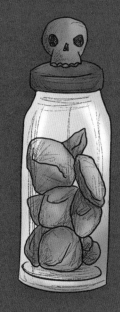
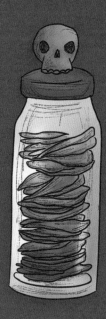

很多人头痛或者生病时都会吃药。不过，你知道吗？制作药品这门"艺术"可以追溯到几千年前！翻开这本书，你会发现，在面对种种疾病时，有的疗法大胆新颖，有的让人恶心，还有一些则充满智慧！

- 把毒蛇泡在酒里制成蛇酒，可以缓解疲劳、治疗脱发
- 蜗牛黏液可用来治疗烧伤，烤小猫咪用来医治黄疸
- 嚼柳树皮可以镇痛，还可以治疗疟疾

　　……

这本书还会探索：几百年前人们如何使用草药治病？保罗·埃尔利希的"神奇子弹"如何治愈致命梅毒？蟑螂、鲇鱼、青蛙自身会产生什么样的抗生素？除此之外，还有很多天然（以及其他）疗法，科学家们从未停止探索的脚步！

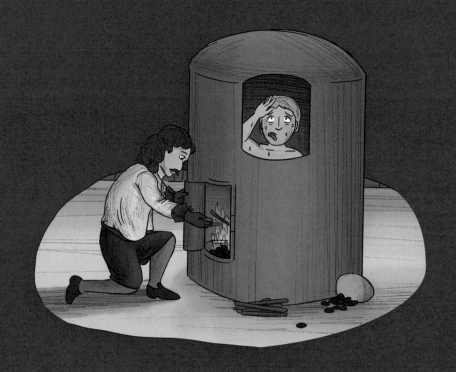

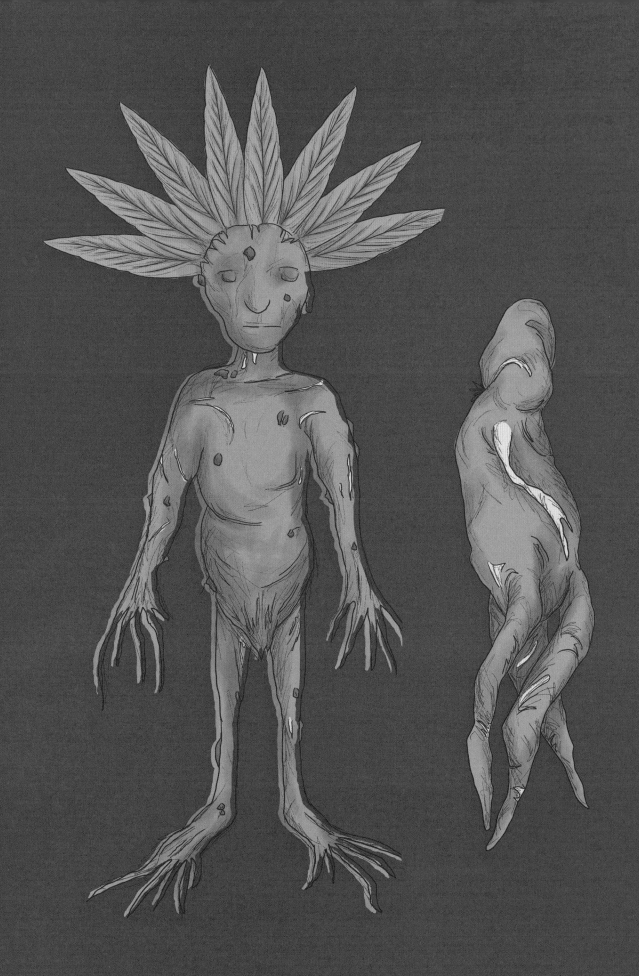

目录

写在前面

　　人们生病之后，需要正确用药才能缓解病情。但是，如何确定哪种药管用呢？从古至今，医生们一直都因这个问题头疼不已。通过这本书，我们可以了解到医生们在用药治病过程中的一些天才想法，当然也会看到一些糟糕透顶的失败案例。

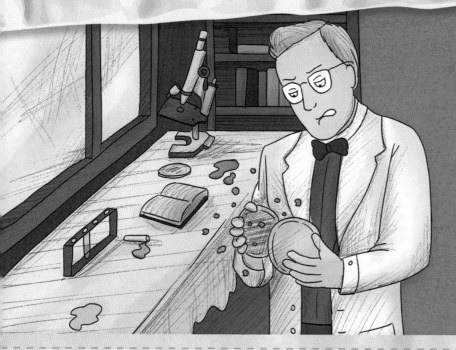

杀菌类药物

　　一些药物通过抑制病菌感染来帮助人们恢复健康。比如说，抗生素就是用来杀死或攻击致病细菌的。但抗生素只对细菌起作用，如果要对付病毒，就得使用专门的抗病毒药物。

调节型药物

　　有时候，我们的身体会产生过多的某类化学物质，而有时又会极度缺乏一些化学物质。因此，制药师们研制了一些药物，或是可以替代人体中缺乏的化学物质，或是可以在身体产生过多的化学物质时，抑制该物质的生成。例如，糖尿病患者通过注射外来胰岛素（过去往往从猪的胰腺中提取）来替代自身无法分泌的胰岛素。

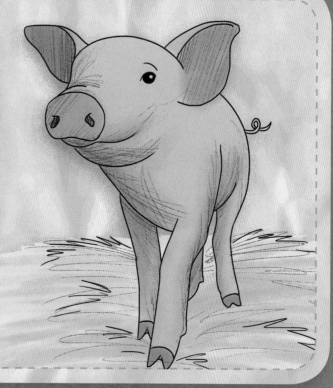

缓解症状类药物

有些药物的作用不是治愈疾病，而仅仅是缓解一些症状，让病人感觉好受些。比如，止痛剂可以缓解头痛和嗓子痛；乳膏能够缓解皮肤瘙痒。

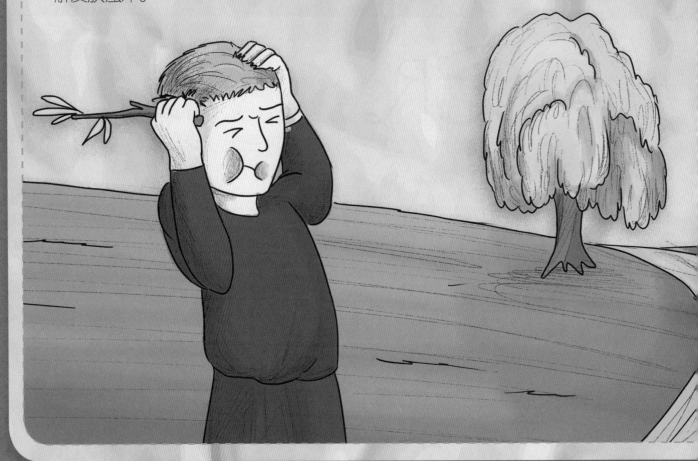

规模庞大的制药业

据说，美国的全民用药量差不多相当于全世界其他地区人们用药量的总和。美国人每年购买和使用的药物价值高达3,000多亿美元！换句话说，每个美国人每年要在药物上花费1,000美元左右。看来他们要么很健康，要么病得很厉害……

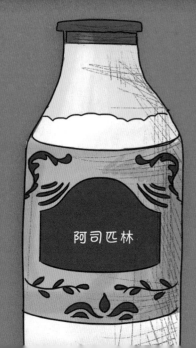

阿司匹林

古代医学

许多药草和自然物质本身就具有治疗功能。但人们很久以前就知道，以特定方法制备或混合这些天然药材，可以收到更好的疗效。这些古老的药物配制术可以追溯到古埃及时期，甚至更早。

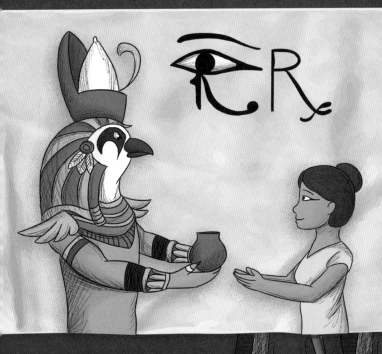

药剂学之父

古埃及人认为药剂学起源于太阳神何露斯。何露斯在一场史诗般的战斗中失去了一只眼睛，但月神透特治好了这只眼睛。如今，药剂师会在药方上写下"Rx"这个符号。有人认为这是古时候"何露斯之眼"的标志，还有人认为它只是中世纪时"处方"一词对应的拉丁语的简略表达。

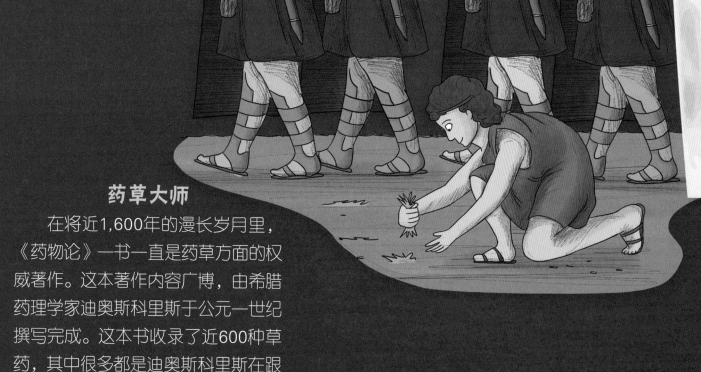

药草大师

在将近1,600年的漫长岁月里，《药物论》一书一直是药草方面的权威著作。这本著作内容广博，由希腊药理学家迪奥斯科里斯于公元一世纪撰写完成。这本书收录了近600种草药，其中很多都是迪奥斯科里斯在跟随罗马军队征战欧洲时发现的。

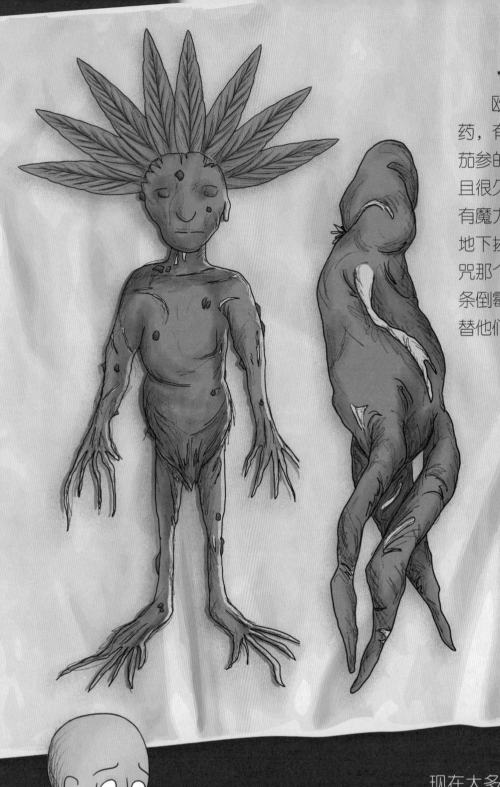

会尖叫的植物根

欧茄参的根是一味强效药，有致幻和催眠的功效。欧茄参的根部呈小小的人形，并且很久以来，人们都认为它拥有魔力。有人说如果谁把它从地下拔出来，它就会尖叫着诅咒那个人。因此，人们会把一条倒霉的狗绑在欧茄参上，代替他们去把根部拔出来。

以底为"口"

现在大多数药物都是口服的。但是，很久以前，一些医生想出了从身体另一端给药的办法。说白了就是医生往病人肛门里插一根管子，也就是"灌肠管"，然后连接另一根管子灌入药物。现在，医生们仍会使用这种方法，将其称为"灌肠法"。

中医古方

中国人有从自然界中寻找药物的古老传统，不仅使用药草，还会用各种匪夷所思的东西入药，包括蝎子尾部的毒针和蜈蚣。

永生不死！

中国的炼丹术士们苦苦寻找能让人长生不死的灵丹妙药，长达数个世纪。传说中一个叫魏伯阳的道士成功炼制出了"永生药"。这个传说还提到，上古的帝王黄帝找到了这种药，得以长生不死。

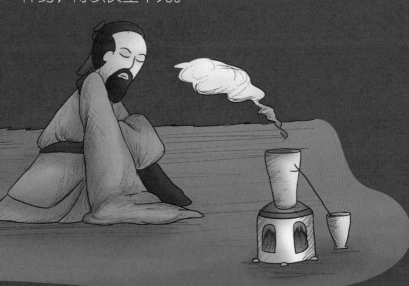

疗病之针

针灸是把一些尖针刺入皮肤。哎哟，好疼！这些针用来刺激人体中可促进病症痊愈的通路——"经络"，从而达到治病的目的。针灸疗法在中国已有2,000多年的历史，欧洲人在很早以前可能也对这种疗法有了认识。冰人奥茨死于5,000多年前，尸体被冻在山上的冰雪中，他身上的刺青似乎就标记了针灸的经络之处。

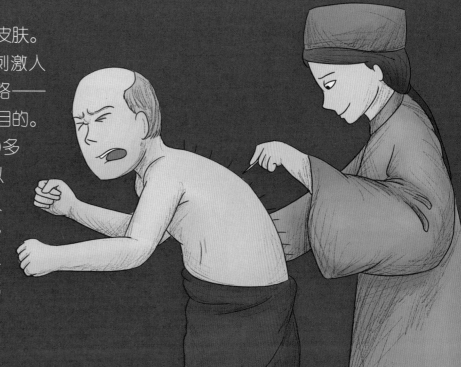

会蜇人的药！

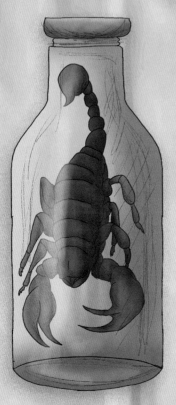

大部分人都会对蝎子退避三舍。要是被它们尾部的毒针蜇一下，会非常疼，甚至会因此丧命。但是，中国人一直认为炮制的蝎子（中药名"全蝎"）可以治愈抽搐、头痛和肿胀。但这也许是因为一看到要用蝎子治病，病人就会大喊："我好了！"

蛇酒

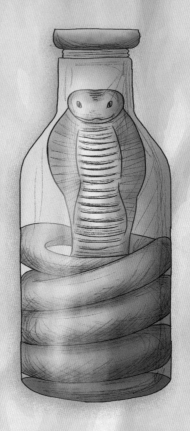

如果你觉得有点累，或者正在掉头发，根据古代中医疗法，你需要喝蛇酒滋补。蛇酒的制作方法是将毒蛇放在黄酒里浸泡。最早在将近2,800年前就有人喝蛇酒了。

海马杀手

海马是美丽的海洋生物，有灭绝的危险。但那些信奉中医的人每年要购买2,500万只海马。他们相信，海马干可以治疗肾疾、气喘、胃痛，以及许多其他病症。

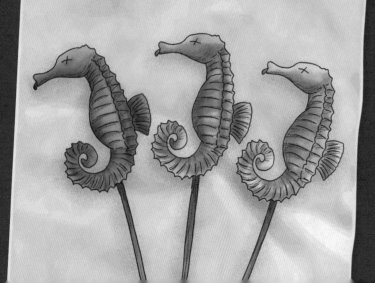

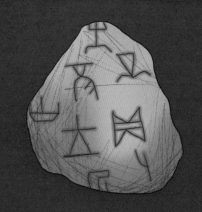

龙骨

在中国，人们常常把古代动物的骨骼化石称作"龙骨"。将这些骨骼化石磨成粉制成中药，可用于治疗心脏疾病、除烦热。在古代中国，龙骨也被称作"甲骨"。人们会在这些甲骨上刻画文字，向神灵卜问吉凶。

早期化学药物

大部分现代药物并不是由药草制成的，而是由化学制品合成而来。对此，我们应该感谢古代伊斯兰世界的科学家，才华横溢的查比尔·伊本·赫扬就是其中的一位先驱。查比尔也被人叫作格伯，1,300年前可能生活在库费（今属伊拉克）。

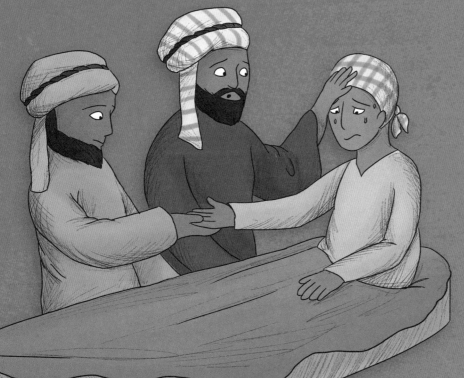

临床问诊

为了获得化学药物的正确配比方式，伊斯兰医生认为应该花时间对每位病人进行诊视，尽可能全面地了解病人的发病症状与个体特征。

吃了毒药会发生什么？

据说，查比尔掌握了当时所有已知毒药的化学特性。在他的名作《毒药之书》中，他介绍了几百种有毒物质以及它们在人体中的化学反应。他还在书中介绍了一些解毒药，并现场展示了它们发挥作用的过程。

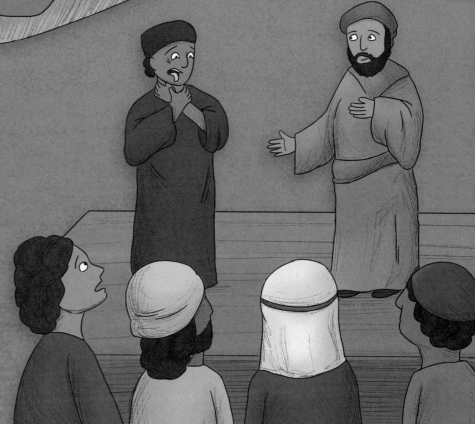

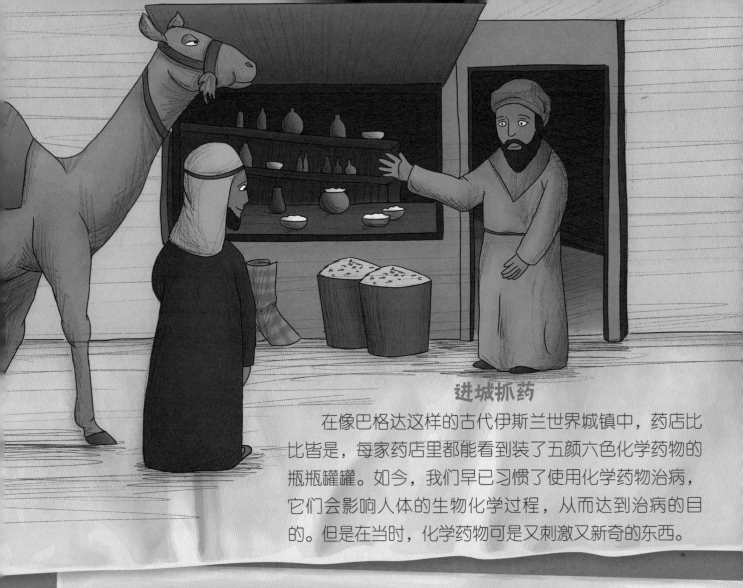

进城抓药

在像巴格达这样的古代伊斯兰世界城镇中，药店比比皆是，每家药店里都能看到装了五颜六色化学药物的瓶瓶罐罐。如今，我们早已习惯了使用化学药物治病，它们会影响人体的生物化学过程，从而达到治病的目的。但是在当时，化学药物可是又刺激又新奇的东西。

夫人，来点毒药?

许多药物含有致命毒素，比如茛菪、毒参和龙葵。这并不是说古代的配药师要用这些药物杀死病人。事实上，他们发现了一个关键问题：用药控制好剂量很重要。服用小剂量的某些毒药可以有效镇痛或促进睡眠。但配药师们并不一定总能调对剂量。调不对的话……拜拜了您嘞！

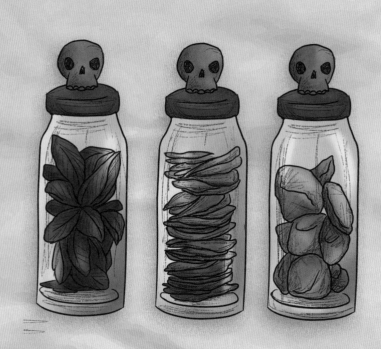

煺毛猫头鹰和烤小猫咪

中世纪的时候，只有非常非常富有的人家才请得起医生诊病。大多数人要是生病了，只能去找配药师。配药师相当于今天的药剂师，他们不仅会告诉你生了什么病，还会拿出自己的治病偏方。

保密的药方

配药师的药店里堆满了各式各样的神秘罐子和奇怪药材。他们喜欢对配方保密，因此会故意让一些药材看上去不知为何物……尽管如此，还是有一些药材可以被辨认出来，比如煺毛后煮熟的猫头鹰（治疗痛风）、刺猬油（治疗咽喉发炎）、蜗牛黏液（治疗烧伤）和烤小猫咪（治疗黄疸）。

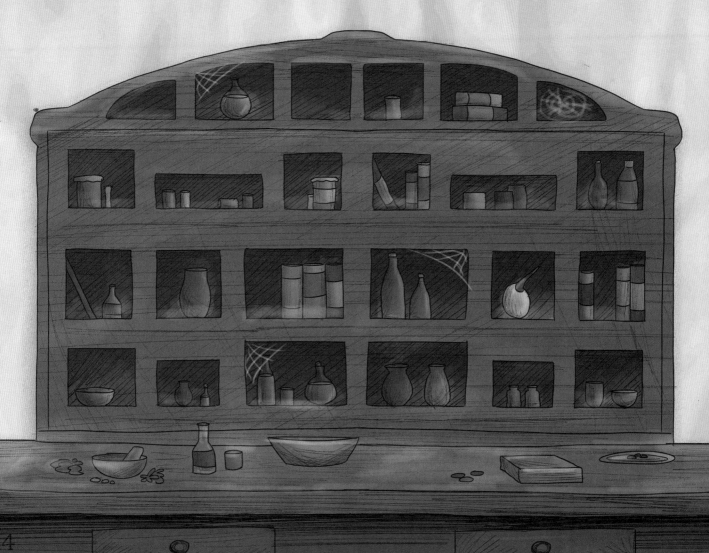

配药方法

配药师为了配制药物，会用天平称量出选好的配料，之后将干燥的配料放进一个叫作"研钵"的结实的碗形容器中，用叫作"杵"的研磨棒磨成粉末。配药师还会用一种叫作"蒸馏釜"的壶形容器提纯和浓缩液体。

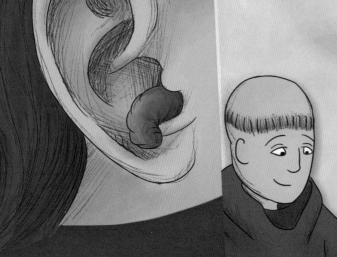

耳朵里的也是"宝"

人身体上脱落的每样东西，似乎也都可以入药，比如毛发、指甲、口水（治疗皮肤过敏）、死皮……如果你头痛得厉害，有的配药师会给你推荐一种把耳屎跟泥和在一起配成的药物，通常做成药膏敷用，似乎疗效不错。

吃屁屁还是喝尿？

有些配药师开的药方非常吓人。如果你喉咙疼痛，他们可能会为你配一勺掺了些蜂蜜的狗屎或婴儿屁屁，让你服下。请注意，如果你背疼，他们会给你一杯掺有牛胆汁、药草和动物板油的尿液让你喝下。而如果发起烧来，你可能需要喝猪尿……

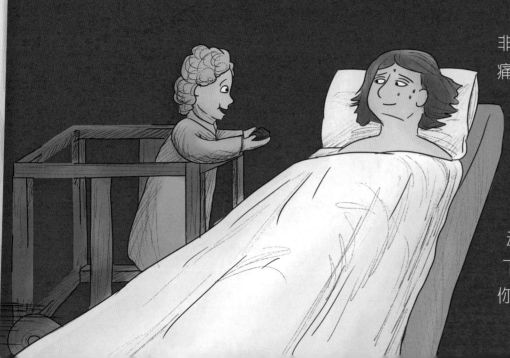

15

绿色药用植物

配药师使用的化学制品和异国药材很难获取，十分昂贵。所以，几个世纪以来，大部分人都是依靠药草来制药。这些药用植物可以从野外采到，也可以种在"药园"里。

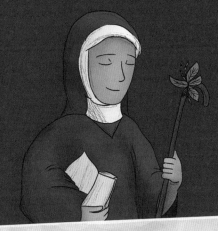

希尔德加德修女的药草

公元12世纪，德国宾根的修女希尔德加德写出了草药学最有名的著作之一。此外，她还是已知最早的作曲家之一。希尔德加德修女信奉"绿色的力量"，她使用植物和药草治愈了多种疾病，著作至今仍被人用作参考。

药用植物园

修道院纷纷修建药用植物园，不仅种植各种用于治疗疾病的药草，还提供一些用于食物调味和染色的草本植物。植物园里分区种植着不同植物，有的用来治疗咳嗽、感冒，有的可治疗肝病和膀胱部位病症，还有一些可助消化，缓解头痛、焦虑和抑郁，林林总总，不一而足。

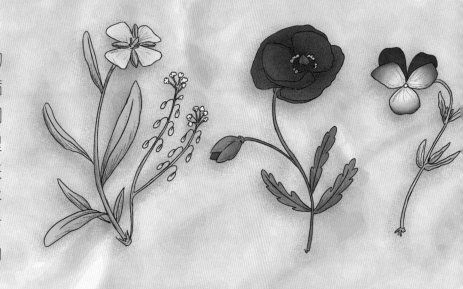

"无所不能"的牛蒡

1653年，尼古拉斯·卡尔佩珀撰写了另一部草药学巨著。但即便是这样一位大学者，也会有一些稀奇古怪的想法。他认为，牛蒡这种药草可以防止放屁、预防狂犬病，还能治愈蛇咬伤。他甚至认为，女性将牛蒡戴在头上可以治疗子宫脱垂……

以形补形

古时候人们很难知道什么东西能治什么病，所以很多人信奉"以形补形说"。

这一学说认为，植物和食物可以治疗身体中跟它们长得像的器官的病症。如此看来，蘑菇切片长得像耳朵，因此肯定有助于改善听力。

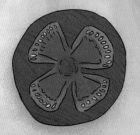
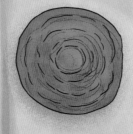
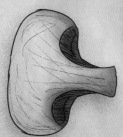
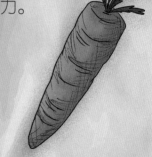

西红柿片——治疗心脏疾病　　胡萝卜片——明目　　蘑菇片——改善听力　　整根胡萝卜——有益鼻子

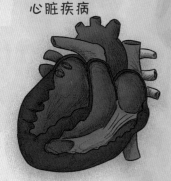
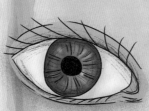
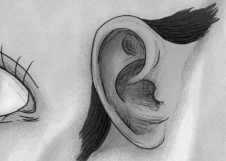
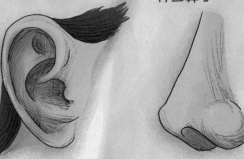

"药到病除"的女巫

在很多乡村里，如果有人生病了，村民会去找女巫看病，因为女巫对治病的药草无所不知。对一些人来说，女巫只是能给人治病、头脑聪明的年长妇女。而在另一些人眼里，女巫拥有法术，令人畏惧，还为恶魔效劳。

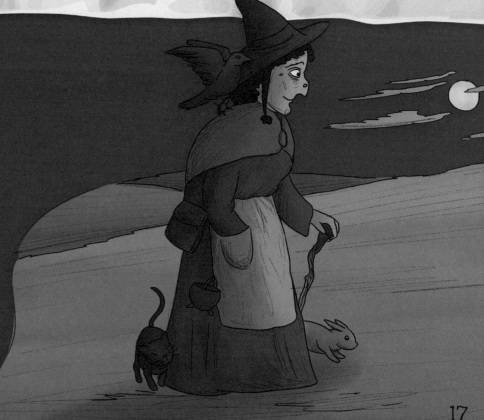

17

柳树的神奇功效

如果有人头痛得厉害，或者其他地方疼痛，他们都会服用阿司匹林或其他止痛药。但一开始并不是这样的……

让人抓狂的树皮

阿司匹林由化学物质水杨酸合成而来。水杨酸以某种形式天然存在于柳树的树皮、香桃木、绣线菊属植物中。但是从这些树中提取水杨酸却是一件让人十分头疼的事……

驯服缠人的"病蛇"

寒热病（可能是疟疾）曾经是一种十分可怕的病症，人们把它形容为一条会紧紧缠住你身体的蛇！嚼金鸡纳树的树皮对治疗寒热病很管用，但在英格兰并不容易找到这种树皮。1758年，牛津郡教区牧师爱德华·斯通注意到，柳树的树皮尝起来有点儿像金鸡纳树的树皮。他让几位寒热病患者试用了这种树皮，发现他们马上感觉好多了。

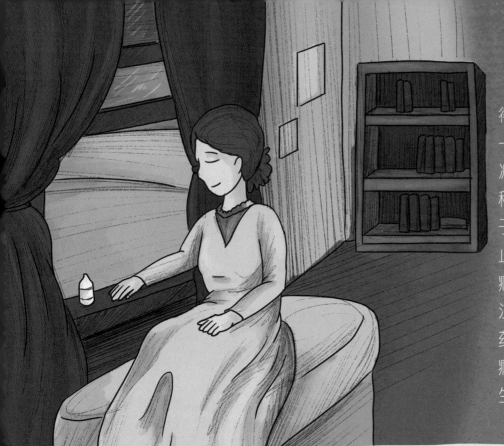

令人上瘾的鸦片酊

19世纪，如果病人觉得哪儿疼，医生就会给他开一瓶鸦片酊。这种药当然会减轻疼痛，但它同时也是一种易成瘾的烈性药物，类似于海洛因（海洛因曾被用作止痛药，但因具有极强的成瘾性，已被禁止使用，译注）。因此，许多吃了这种药的人患上了严重的药物上瘾症，包括许多仅仅想缓解生理期疼痛的女子。

阿司匹林

柳树皮中可以缓解疼痛的成分是一种名为水杨酸的化学物质。但水杨酸会对人的肠胃造成损伤。19世纪90年代，拜耳公司的科学家们对水杨酸进行了改进，降低了它的副作用，合成出"伤害小、疗效大"的神奇药物——阿司匹林。

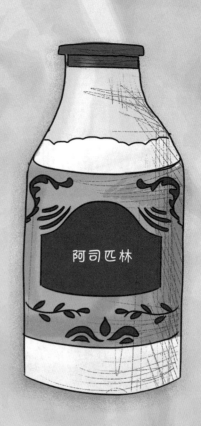

阿司匹林

治愈梅毒的 "神奇子弹"

梅毒是一种曾经肆虐欧洲的可怕疾病，人们一度对它无计可施，直到后来一位德国医生找到了一种化学药物。这种药物既可以杀死梅毒病原体，又不会伤害病人。对他来说，这就是传说中只会杀死致病病菌的"神奇子弹"。

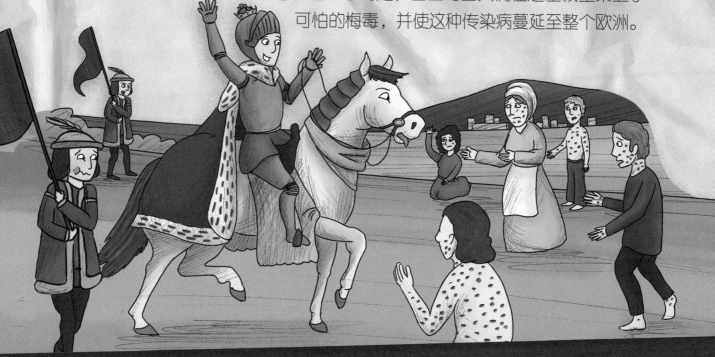

赢了战争，得了梅毒

1495年，法国国王查理八世率领军队征服了意大利那不勒斯，率军入城的国王当时可谓是春风得意。但不幸的是，国王的士兵们在这座城里染上了可怕的梅毒，并使这种传染病蔓延至整个欧洲。

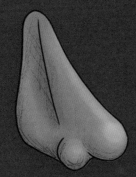

鼻子的"天敌"

梅毒通常并不会直接致人死亡，但染上梅毒后症状十分可怕。梅毒会使人全身长满脓疱，发出难闻的气味，因此也叫"大痘病"。梅毒还会导致患者的鼻子腐烂，因此许多梅毒患者不得不戴上人工鼻子。梅毒还会导致患者精神失常。

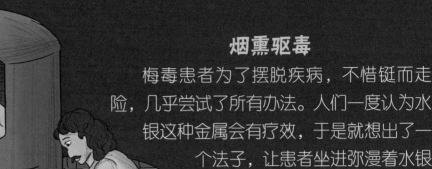

烟熏驱毒

梅毒患者为了摆脱疾病，不惜铤而走险，几乎尝试了所有办法。人们一度认为水银这种金属会有疗效，于是就想出了一个法子，让患者坐进弥漫着水银蒸气的铁箱里接受熏蒸。但是水银本身也有毒，它的副作用使病人极其痛苦难过，甚至丧命。

疑似受害者——
耳聋的天才作曲家

德国天才作曲家路德维希·范·贝多芬（1770—1827）随着年纪渐长出现耳聋，这让他的音乐创作变得无比困难。人们怀疑他的耳聋可能是由梅毒引起的。历史上其他可能感染过梅毒的名人还有英格兰国王亨利八世、德国独裁者阿道夫·希特勒以及俄国作家列夫·托尔斯泰。

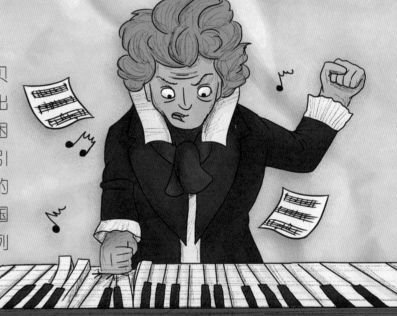

直击靶心——"梅毒克星"诞生

德国科学家保罗·埃尔利希（1854—1915）认为，如果细菌能被某种染料染色，那么也可能被这种染料杀死，就像遇到"神奇子弹"一样。他和同事尝试了几百种染料，终于找到了对梅毒病原体起作用的染料。他们以此为基础研制出了洒尔佛散，这是第一种可以有效治疗梅毒的药物。

救命的霉菌

发霉的食物看上去很恶心，你也不会想吃它。但是，苏格兰科学家亚历山大·弗莱明正是在霉菌中发现了令人惊叹的药物——青霉素。

危险的球菌

金黄色葡萄球菌（以下简称"金葡菌"）是世界上最常见的细菌之一。全球每五个人中可能就有一个人的皮肤表面和鼻子中携带金葡菌。携带金葡菌不一定会引起感染，但一旦感染，病人的病情就会很严重。许多疾病都与金葡菌有关，比如脑膜炎、肺炎、骨髓炎（一种骨科疾病）、流感、疖肿等等。

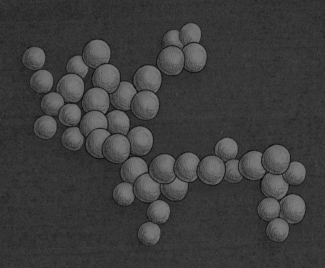

因祸得福——发现青霉素

1928年，弗莱明在实验室中研究收集在培养皿中的金葡菌，中途外出度假。他度假回来后，发现一些培养皿已经发霉了。接下来他又注意到，在有霉菌生长的地方，金葡菌全都死掉了。这让他意识到这些霉菌含有能杀死金葡菌的天然物质，他把这种物质命名为"青霉素"。

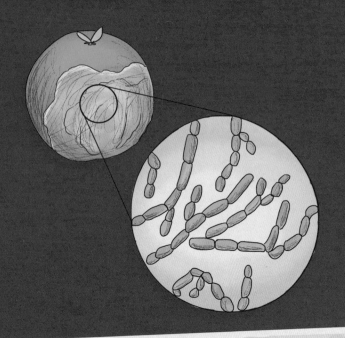

青霉素是什么？

弗莱明在特异青霉（一种青霉菌，译注）中找到了青霉素。特异青霉是一种真菌。与所有霉菌一样，特异青霉也呈丝状生长，这种丝叫作"菌丝"。特异青霉会生出微小的孢子（类似于种子），在空气中广泛散播。橘子发霉以后表面会长出绿色的毛，这些绿毛就是指状青霉。而蓝干酪中的蓝色纹理则是罗克福尔青霉。

登陆战士的"回魂丹"

科学家霍华德·弗洛里和恩斯特·钱恩将弗莱明发现的青霉素转变成药品，可以拯救成千上万人的生命。这两位科学家找到了大批量生产青霉素的方法，使青霉素可以用来治疗被感染的伤口。二战时，青霉素拯救了无数在1944年诺曼底登陆中受伤的军人的生命。

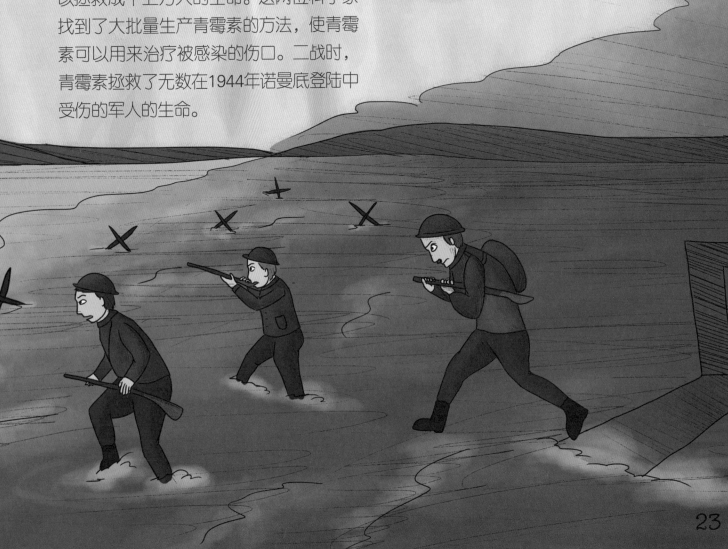

自然界的病菌杀手

自弗莱明发现青霉素以来，科学家们已经发现了数千种抗生素，即专门对抗细菌的药物。现在使用的大部分抗生素完全是人工合成的，但是和青霉素一样，很多抗生素最初也是从自然界中发现的。比如，四环素和链霉素这两种抗生素的发现就来源于细菌。自然界中有很多可供药物研制人员开发新药的抗生素类物质。下面我们就来看看，科学家寻找抗生素的地方哪些最为匪夷所思……

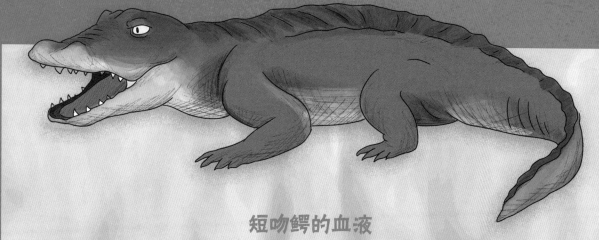

短吻鳄的血液

科学家们发现一种令他们感到困惑的现象：短吻鳄间相互搏斗后，看上去受了重伤，但它们的伤口并没有感染。经过研究，他们发现，短吻鳄的血液中含有天然抗生素，能够有效抵御多种感染的侵害。

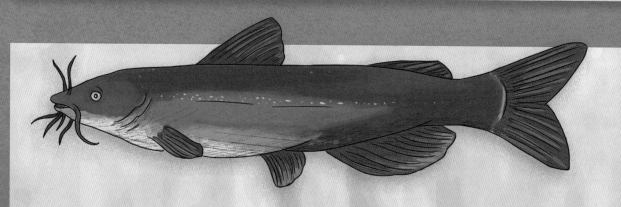

鲇鱼的黏液

鲇鱼受伤后似乎也不会感染，科学家们找到了原因。鲇鱼的身体被一层富含抗生素的黏液包裹，黏液中的抗生素可以有效杀死侵害肺部的肺炎克雷伯氏菌以及大肠杆菌等病菌。

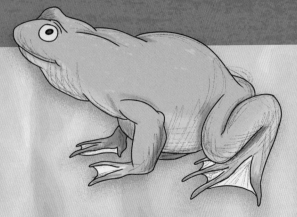

神奇的青蛙皮肤

青蛙能够存活在许多生物无法生存的水体里。现在，科学家们找到了原因之一：青蛙皮肤中含有近100种杀菌物质。不过这些物质中的大多数对人体有害，因此科学家们必须要找到一种方法，在不伤害人类自身的前提下利用这些杀菌物质。

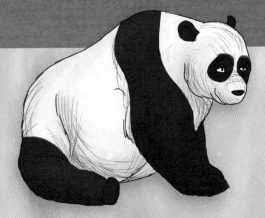

熊猫血液中的高效"杀手"

最厉害的抗生素之一，抗菌肽–AM，存在于熊猫的血液之中。与其他抗生素相比，它只需要几分之一的时间便可以杀灭病菌。但由于熊猫是珍稀动物，科学家只能通过人工合成熊猫血液进行抗菌肽–AM的实验研究。

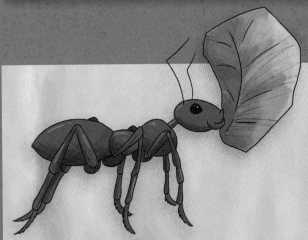

切叶蚁的多重自卫"武器"

切叶蚁搬运叶子的超强能力广为人知，但它们抵御病菌的本事也不小。科学家们发现，切叶蚁的身体可以产生多种化学物质，能够合力对抗细菌和真菌的攻击，这和医生在治疗严重感染时采用多种药物、多管齐下是一个道理。

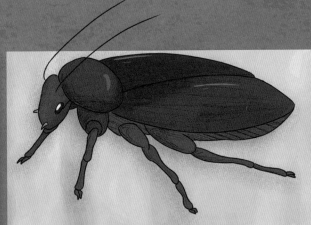

蟑螂脑组织中的"宝贝"

压碎的蟑螂脑组织中含有九种不同的抗生素。科学家们正试着从中找出一些抗生素来治疗大肠杆菌感染，甚至耐甲氧西林金黄色葡萄球菌（MRSA）感染。MRSA是一种超级金葡菌，对一般抗生素都有耐药性。

血糖与糖尿病

糖尿病患者的血糖难以保持在较低水平，这个问题出在患者体内的化学物质胰岛素上面。胰岛素本可以调节血糖，但糖尿病患者体内的胰岛素出了问题（胰岛素分泌缺陷或生物作用受损，译注），无法调节血糖。因此糖尿病患者需要定期注射胰岛素。

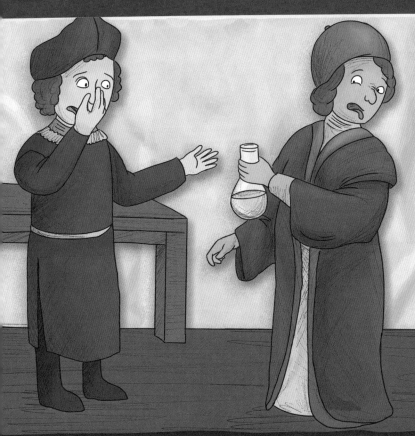

有甜味的尿液

中世纪时，许多医生仅仅知道如何诊断糖尿病——尝一尝病人的尿液。如果尿液尝起来有甜味，那么病人就得了糖尿病。但是，他们对治疗糖尿病却无计可施。有人建议喝红酒，有人认为进食大量酸味食物有用，甚至还有人认为骑马能治疗糖尿病！

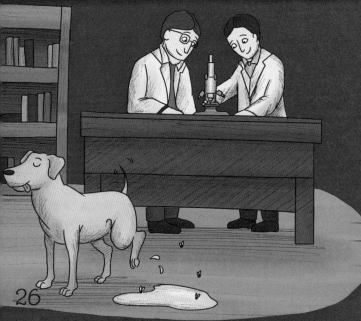

胰岛素的发现

1889年，德国科学家奥斯卡·闵可夫斯基和约瑟夫·冯·梅林为了研究消化功能，切除了一只狗的胰腺。之后，他们观察到这只狗的尿液引来了苍蝇吸食，从而发现尿液带有甜味，因此二人意识到胰腺能够控制血糖水平。1921年，加拿大人弗雷德里克·班廷和美国人查尔斯·H.贝斯特进一步发现，胰腺通过产生胰岛素控制血糖水平。

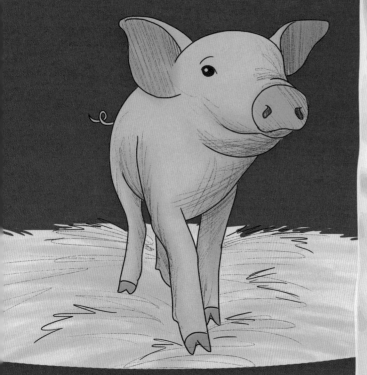

生产胰岛素的"细菌工厂"

20世纪70年代，科学家们找到了以细菌为"工厂"生产人胰岛素的方法。他们将表达人胰岛素的基因拼接到大肠杆菌的DNA分子中，然后将大肠杆菌置于大桶中进行繁殖。此时，大肠杆菌就会按照新的基因指令进行繁殖，从而产生大量人胰岛素。目前，这是获取治疗糖尿病所需的胰岛素的主要方法。

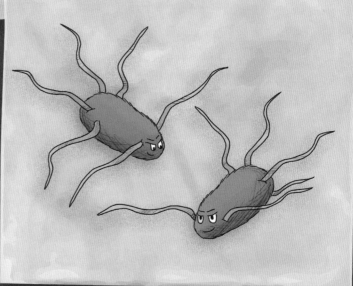

糖尿病患者的"救星"
——猪和牛

对于糖尿病的治疗来说，发现胰岛素是一个重大突破。胰岛素可以从肉用猪和牛的胰腺中提取。提取的猪或牛的胰岛素再经过提纯，即可注射进糖尿病患者体内，控制患者的血糖水平。

防止"恶魔出笼"

潘多拉是神话中的女孩，她出于好奇打开了魔盒，放出了战争、疾病等会伤害人类的恶魔。一些科学家担心，为了合成胰岛素而培育的转基因细菌会有泄漏和传播的风险——就像打开了潘多拉的魔盒。1975年，在一次大会上，科学家们一致同意永远不使用致病细菌，而且所有研究工作都要在绝对安全的房间中进行。

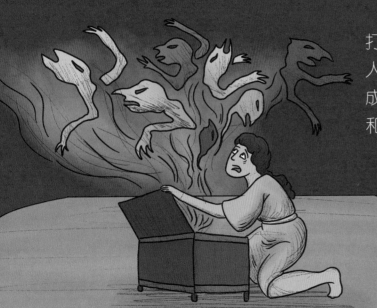

回看药物发展史

人类所服用的药物，从几千年前的简易药草，到今天大规模生产的化学药物，经历了漫长的发展历程。以下是药物发展史中一些具有里程碑意义的事件。

约1520年 证实剂量的作用

德裔瑞士籍学者帕拉切尔苏斯有点像个怪胎，总是搞一些神秘兮兮的东西。但也正是他，证实了服用药物（包括毒药）必须剂量适当才能获得理想的治疗效果。

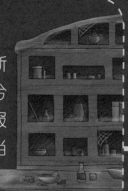

公元前1000年

1000年

约公元前2800年 神农尝百草

神农是中国神话中的皇帝，他品尝了数百种药草，亲自验证了它们的药效，为流传至今的中国传统医学奠定了基础。

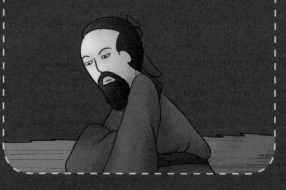

约公元800年 《毒药之书》写成

波斯化学家查比尔·伊本·赫扬撰写了《毒药之书》，这是最早的关于药物化学成分的著作之一。

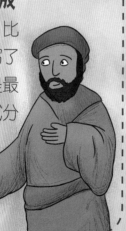

约公元60年 《药物论》问世

希腊医生迪奥斯科里斯写出了五卷本《药物论》，介绍了各类药草和其他一些药用物质的疗效。

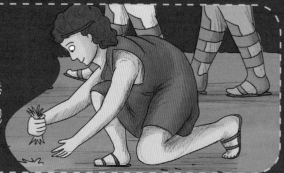

1899年
阿司匹林诞生

拜耳化工公司研制出了阿司匹林，这是最早的广泛售卖的常规止痛药之一。

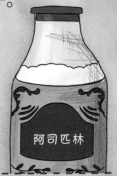

1921年 "甜蜜"的发现

弗雷德里克·班廷、查尔斯·贝斯特和约翰·麦克劳德发现了胰岛素。胰岛素由胰腺分泌，能够控制血糖水平。注射人工胰岛素可以治疗糖尿病。

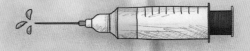

1800年 2000年

1910年
"神奇子弹"研制成功

洒尔佛散是针对致病细菌研制的第一发"神奇子弹"，是第一种能有效治疗梅毒的药品。

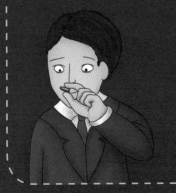

1928年
发现青霉素

苏格兰医生亚历山大·弗莱明在青霉菌中发现了青霉素，这是人类最早发现的天然抗生素之一。

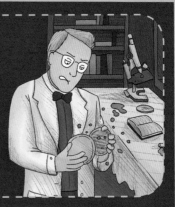

1948年
抗炎症药物出现

爱德华·肯德尔和菲利普·亨奇发现了皮质类固醇，可以用作消炎药，而风湿病等疾病的主要症状就是炎症。

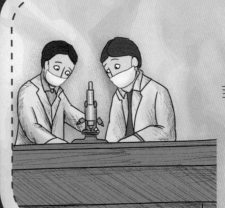

偏方奇药面面观

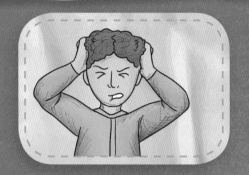

要治疗头痛和精神萎靡，中世纪的草药医生会调配含有药水苏和马鞭草两种药草的药物。现在，科学家们发现，这两种药草中都含有可以缓解偏头痛和抑郁症状的化学成分。

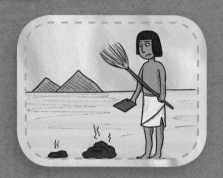

据古代纸莎草纸文献记载，古埃及人会把驴粪、狗粪、瞪羚屎和苍蝇屎用作药物口服。

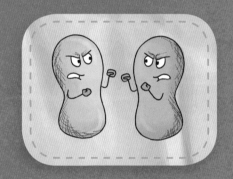

自发现抗生素以来，越来越多的细菌产生了耐药性，这主要是由滥用抗生素造成的。

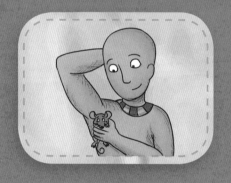

古埃及人把蜥蜴血、死老鼠、泥土和发霉的面包用作治疮的"药膏"。

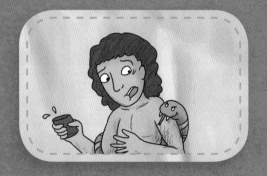

传说古希腊国王米特拉达梯研制了一种可以解百毒的解毒药。罗马人将其制成解毒糖剂，用于治疗各种小病小恙。实际上这种糖剂并不顶用，但直到19世纪末，人们才停止使用这种药。

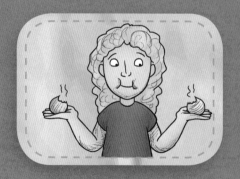

最近，科学家们验证了中世纪时一种治疗眼疾的药物的疗效。这种药由洋葱、大蒜、红酒和公牛胆汁制成，虽然看上去很恶心，但却有着惊人的杀菌效果。

术语表

杵	一种棒状物，配药师用来在研钵中将药物研磨成粉末
灌肠管	自病人肛门插入，用于灌注液体、气体的医用管子
抗生素	对抗细菌的药物
配药师	古代配制、售卖药品的人
青霉素	青霉菌中可以杀死细菌的物质
水杨酸	一种存在于绣线菊属植物和柳树的树皮中的物质，可用于消炎，也可用来合成阿司匹林
细菌	一种单细胞微生物
鸦片酊	一种会使人上瘾的止痛药水，通过将鸦片溶入酒精制成
研钵	配药师用来研磨、混合药物的碗形容器
胰岛素	人体中调节血糖水平的化学物质
"以形补形说"	一种治病理念，认为自然界中与人体器官形状相似的物体可以用来治疗该器官的病症
针灸	一种中国古代就已出现的治疗手法，通过将尖针刺入人体实施治疗
蒸馏釜	配药师用来提纯液体的水壶形容器，有细长的出液管

索引

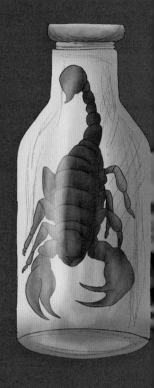

作者简介

约翰·法恩登是位多产的科普图书作家，作品涉及科学、技术和自然领域，包括全球畅销书《放我出去》和《你觉得自己聪明吗？》，并曾五次获得英国皇家学会青少年科学图书奖的提名。

绘者简介

温妮莎·迪安成长于英国布赖顿，从小时候能握住铅笔起就十分热爱绘画。她在19岁生日时收到了一个电子绘画板，便开始尝试电子绘画，从此在这条路上探索不止。

The Grisly History of Medicine

Kill or Cure

Written by John Farndon
Illustrated by Venitia Dean

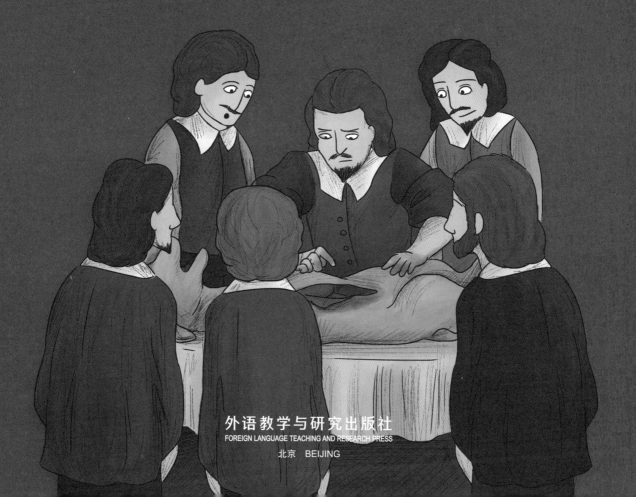

外语教学与研究出版社
FOREIGN LANGUAGE TEACHING AND RESEARCH PRESS
北京 BEIJING

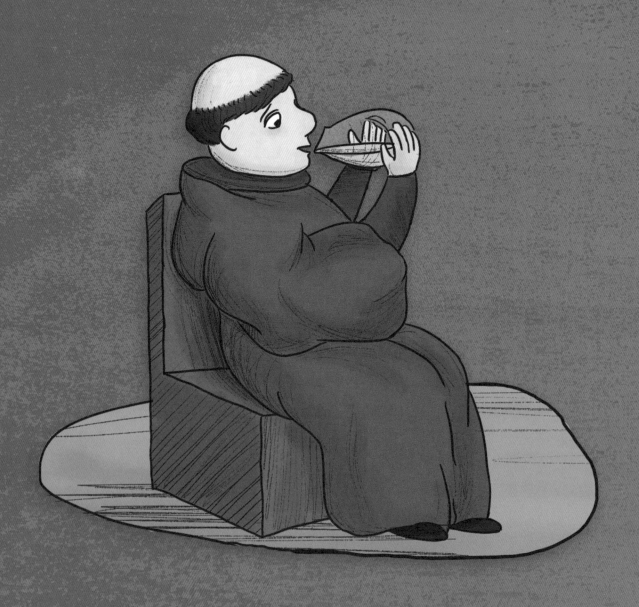

People have always got sick, so they have always needed doctors. But while most doctors tried to help their patients, sometimes their methods were weird, disgusting or even dangerous. Yet this was how modern practices began.

- Noses were rebuilt by attaching the skin from an arm
- The first blood transfusion was between two dogs
- The ancient Chinese immunised against smallpox with powdered pus

  ...

If you're not too squeamish, you'll see barbers doubling up as surgeons, leeches drawing out blood, and corpses being dug up so doctors could study anatomy – along with the first anaesthetics to remove pain, one of medicine's great miracles.

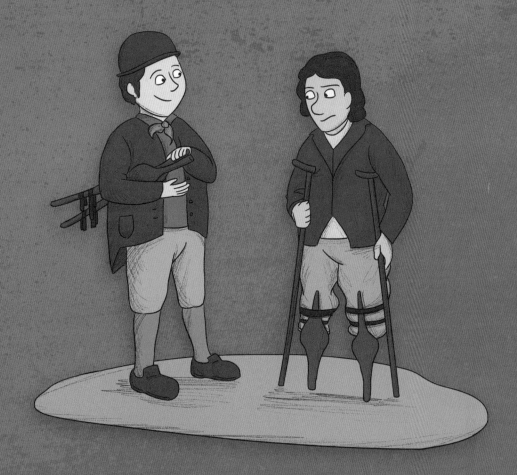

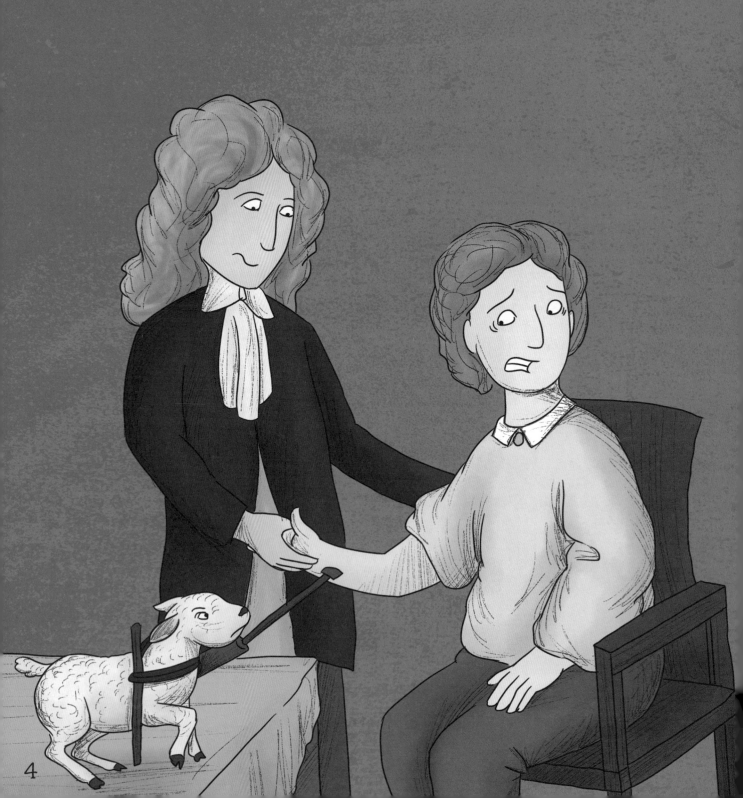

Contents

INTRODUCTION

People have always got sick, so they have always needed doctors. But while most doctors try to make you better, sometimes in the past their methods were weird, yucky or even dangerous. Did you know there were doctors who liked to drink your urine, and others that liked to blow smoke up your rear end? Well, read on...

We need more doctors!

There are about 69 million health workers in the world. The World Health Organization thinks that we really need over 4 million more health workers.

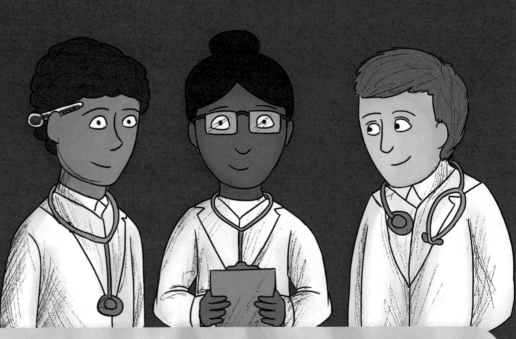

Long training

If you want to be a doctor, you have a lot to learn! It takes ten years on average to train to be a general practitioner (GP). Some specialists have to train for up to 16 years before they are fully qualified.

Lady doctor?

There were women doctors as long ago as the time of Ancient Egypt. But they often had to pretend to be men to be allowed to practise, like Agnodice in Ancient Greece, and the British Army doctor, James Barry (Margaret Ann Bulkley), who lived in the 19th century.

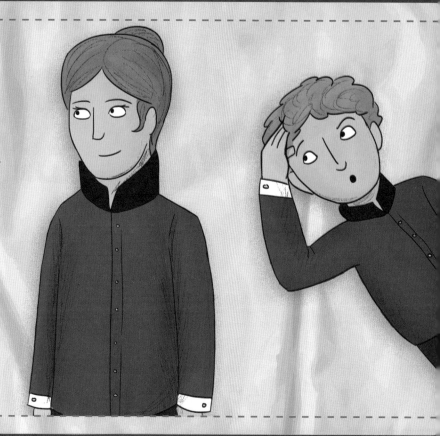

There's money in medicine

In the USA, doctors are generally well paid. One of the best paid are specialists in orthopaedics, who treat bones and muscles. They earn nearly half a million dollars a year.

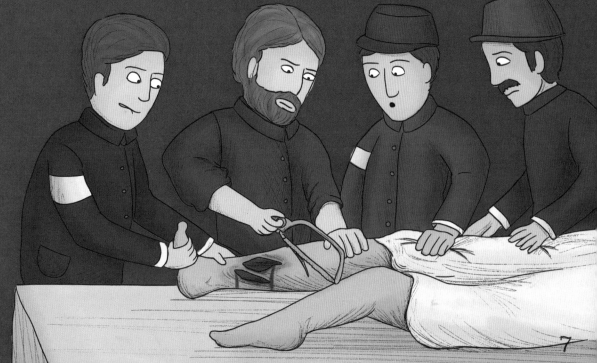

CUTTING AND DRILLING

Today surgery is done with the latest high tech equipment while you're asleep. But the first surgeons cut into you while you lay screaming in agony. Sometimes, though, they might just have saved your life.

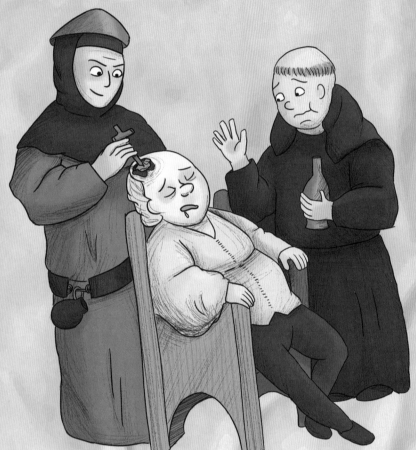

Hole in the head

'Trepanning' dates back about 7,000 years. It involves drilling a large hole in the skull! It sounds unbelievably painful and very dangerous. Yet trepanning was practised right up until a few hundred years ago. No one really knows why. Maybe it was to stop people suffering fits, or to let evil spirits out.

Stitched up!

People were stitching up serious wounds with a needle and thread at least 6,000 years ago. They'd sew the wound together with a bone needle and thread made from animal tendons or plant fibres. Now we call this 'suturing'. Back then they probably just said 'aaagh'!

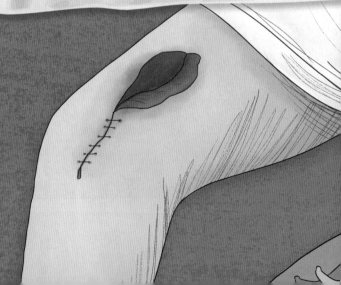

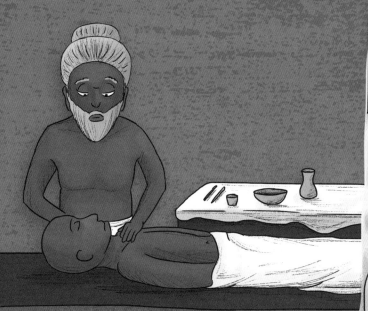

Nose job

One of the earliest known plastic surgeons, Sushruta, lived in India 2,800 years ago. Back then, noses were chopped off as a punishment. So Sushruta developed a line in rebuilding noses. He simply cut a flap from your cheek, then folded it over to make a new nose, holding it in place with stitches until it was properly grafted (attached).

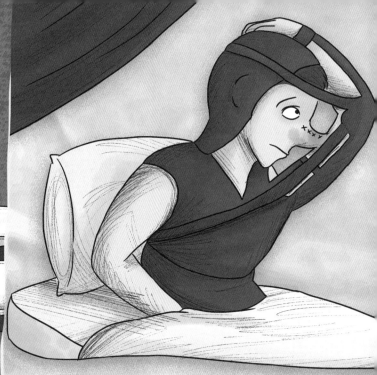

Nose job (No.2)

In 15th-century Italy, if you lost your nose in a sword fight (as many did), you went to Dr Gaspare Tagliacozzi. Tagliacozzi would rebuild your nose for you by grafting skin from your arm. This meant going around with your arm sewn to your nose for months. And it wasn't guaranteed to work.

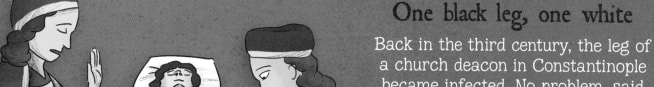

One black leg, one white

Back in the third century, the leg of a church deacon in Constantinople became infected. No problem, said local saints Cosmas and Damian to the deacon, in a dream. They cut off his diseased leg and stitched another in its place, chopped from a newly dead body. But the dead man was black. So when the deacon woke up, he had one black leg and one white! If the story is true, it was the first ever transplant...

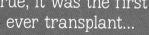

DOCTORS FROM OLD TIMES

In prehistoric times, people relied on magic and traditional knowledge when they fell ill. But most modern doctors try to use scientific knowledge instead. It is said that the first specialist doctors appeared in the time of Ancient Egypt, nearly 5,000 years ago.

Stretched

The Greek doctor Hippocrates (see opposite) invented this device, in which the patient was stretched with ropes tied round their arms and legs. It looks pretty nasty, and it inspired the medieval torture device, the rack. But it was designed to help set broken bones properly – and hospitals still use similar 'traction' devices to relieve pressure on damaged backs.

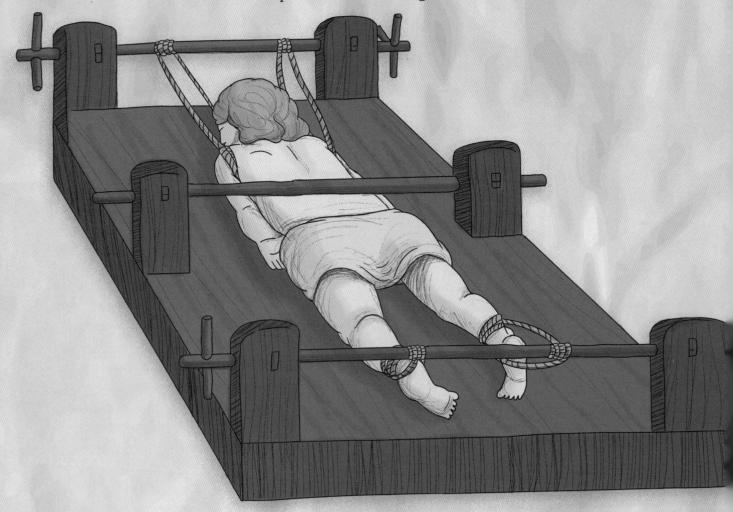

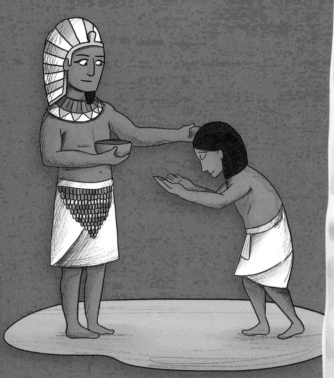

No snakes, please!

Hippocrates lived on the Greek island of Kos about 2,500 years ago. Ancient Greek doctors often killed patients by trying to cure them with snake venom, but Hippocrates knew this was wrong – diseases weren't punishments by the gods but had natural causes. He also said doctors had a duty of care to patients.

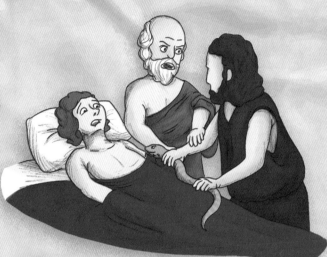

Doctors today still swear a Hippocratic Oath to treat patients well, based on Hippocrates' ideas.

I want my mummy!

It is said that the first known doctor was Imhotep, who lived in Egypt about 4,600 years ago. Apparently he could diagnose and treat about 200 diseases, such as tuberculosis and arthritis. He knew anatomy, too, and maybe even how blood circulates. He was also a brilliant engineer who built pyramids. So if he didn't cure you, he'd give you a good tomb!

Nasty wound, there! Great!

Galen (129 AD–c. 216 AD) was one of the most famous doctors in the Roman Empire. He learnt what bodies are really like from the terrible wounds that gladiators suffered in fights. His knowledge became the basis of medicine for over 1,400 years. Galen boasted, 'I have done as much for medicine as Trajan did for the Roman Empire when he built bridges and roads.'

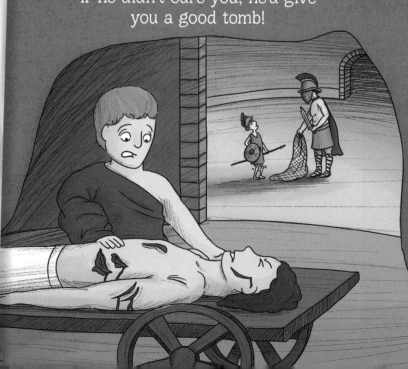

HUMOURS AND MOODS

In Ancient Greece and Rome and in the Middle Ages, doctors thought you have four body fluids called humours – and you get ill when you have too much of one of them. Their treatments were about trying to put the balance right.

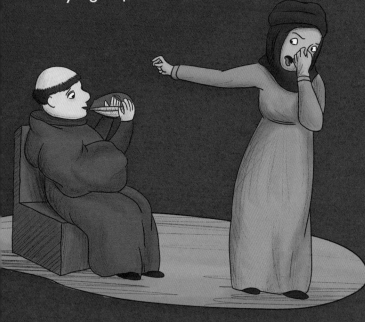

Urine trouble

Some doctors in the Middle Ages thought they could tell what was wrong with you from another body fluid – urine. They didn't just look at its colour. They smelt it, and even tasted it. Yuck! But they knew that a sweet taste meant a patient had diabetes.

The humours were each linked to different nasty fluids that you sometimes cough up. The humours didn't just affect your body, though. They influenced your whole character. And each was linked to a particular season and type of weather.

A Yellow bile

You may vomit up half-digested food with this yellow stomach juice. Yellow bile was linked to problems with the liver. It was also related to a cross and irritable, or passionate, impulsive nature, and to summer and hot, dry weather.

B Blood

You can sometimes cough up blood or have a nosebleed. Blood was linked to problems with the heart. It was also associated with a cheery and hopeful, optimistic and artistic nature, and to spring and warm, moist weather.

C Phlegm

Phlegm is the slimy stuff you cough up or sneeze out when you have a cold. Phlegm was linked to a shy, reserved, caring and thoughtful – and sometimes lazy – nature, and to winter and cold, wet weather.

D Black bile

Black bile is the smelly liquid you can vomit up even when you haven't eaten. It was linked to problems with the spleen. Black bile was associated with a moody and depressed, but rather analytical nature, and to autumn and cold, dry weather.

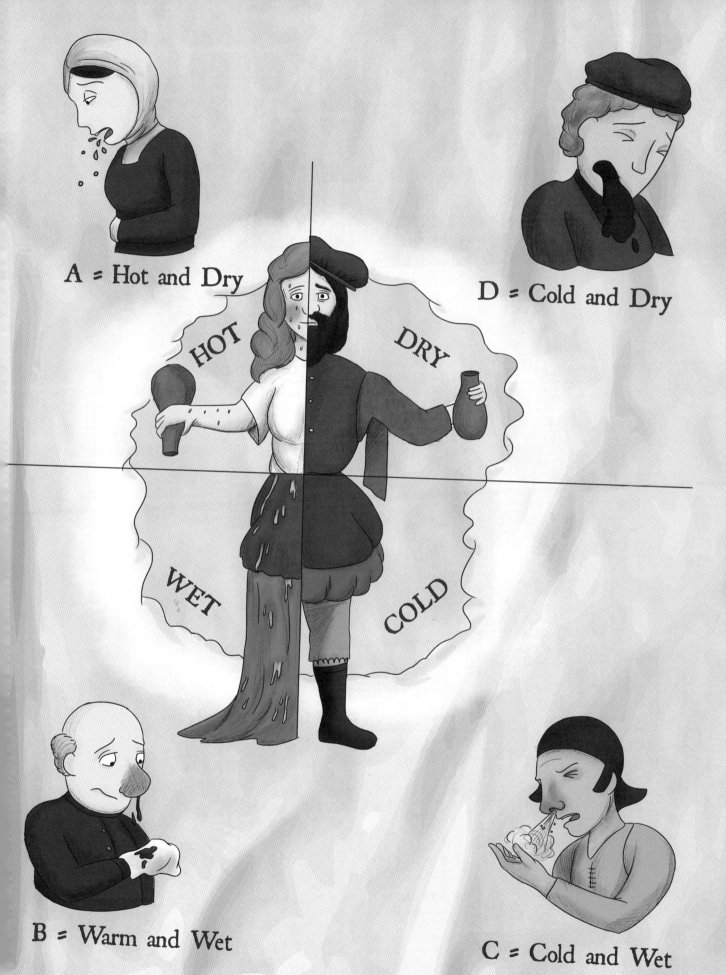

A = Hot and Dry

D = Cold and Dry

HOT

DRY

WET

COLD

B = Warm and Wet

C = Cold and Wet

13

BODY BUTCHERS - THE ANATOMISTS

From the 1500s on, people thought it might help to know where things are actually positioned in our bodies (our anatomy) and how they work (our physiology). But finding out could be a rather nasty business!

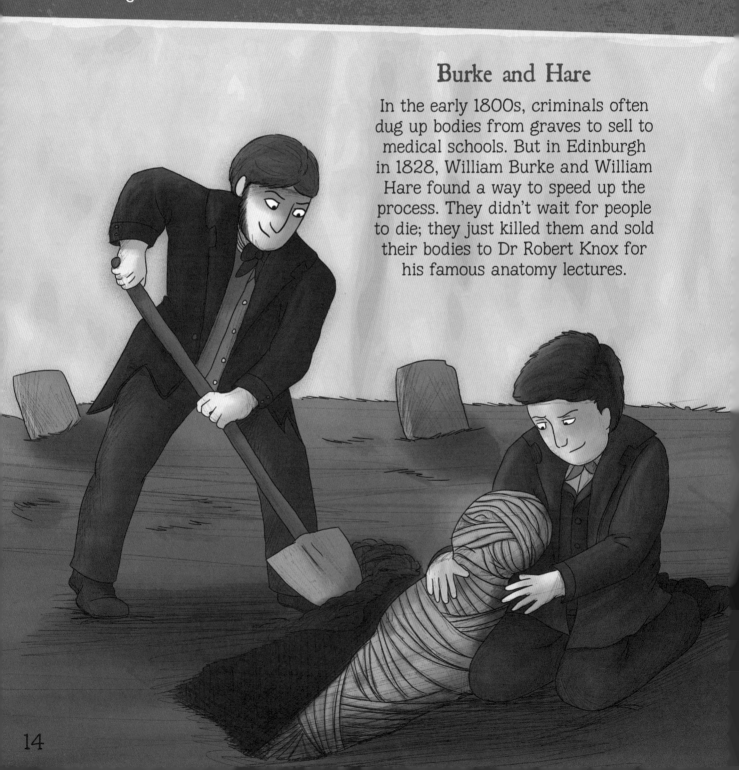

Burke and Hare

In the early 1800s, criminals often dug up bodies from graves to sell to medical schools. But in Edinburgh in 1828, William Burke and William Hare found a way to speed up the process. They didn't wait for people to die; they just killed them and sold their bodies to Dr Robert Knox for his famous anatomy lectures.

Cut up

In the 1530s, Italian doctor Andreas Vesalius realised that the only way to learn about human anatomy was to cut bodies open. He did this to make detailed, accurate drawings of what is inside. Cutting up bodies is called 'dissection'. In 1540, he dissected the body of a criminal in front of a huge audience.

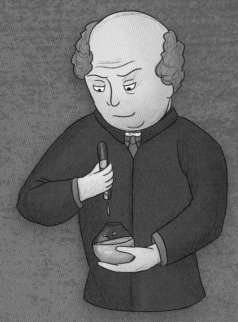

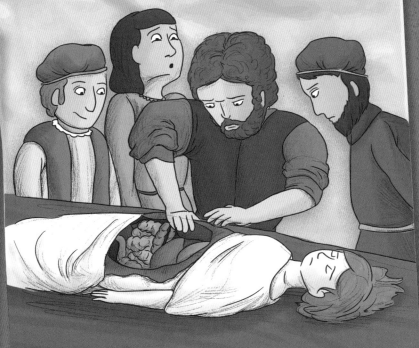

I said half a teaspoon...

German-Swiss doctor Paracelsus (1493–1541) developed the idea that different drugs could be used for different diseases. But he had a strange interest in poisons. When people attacked him for it, he said that poisons are only poisonous if you have a big enough dose. He tested this theory on animals...

Circulation

In the early 1600s, William Harvey showed that blood doesn't just sit in the body, it is pumped round and round by the heart. This was a medical breakthrough. But the way Harvey showed this seems really cruel now. He tied a living dog to a table, then cut it open to show the dog's heart pumping and the blood flowing.

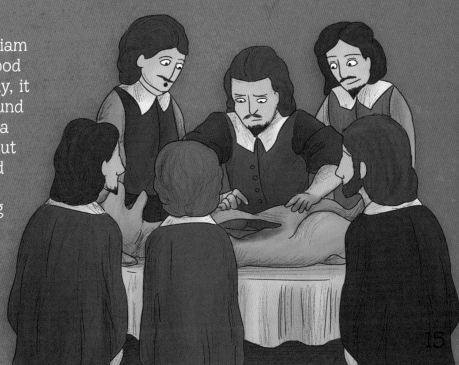

STRANGE TREATMENTS

Next time you complain about having to take medicine when you're ill, just think about what you might have had to go through in the past – anything from being covered in bloodsucking slugs to being cut and made to bleed.

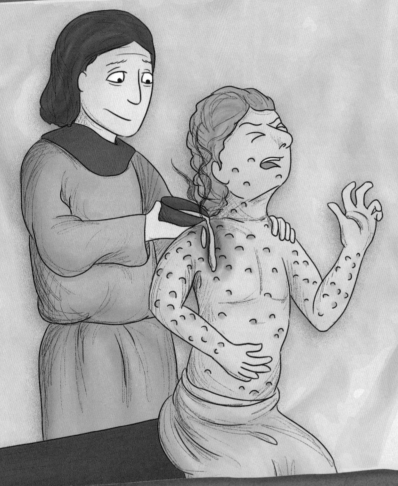

Heavy metal

In the 1490s, the terrible disease syphilis began to spread across Europe. One of its effects was to cover the body in horrible pustules. To treat the disease, doctors spooned the liquid metal mercury on the pustules or made patients sit in a room filled with mercury vapour. But mercury is poisonous and drove patients mad.

Fancy the cupping?

Cupping dates back nearly 5,000 years and is still performed by some people today. It involves heating a cup and pressing it hard onto the skin. The heat creates a suction effect that draws blood to the skin under the cup. The extra blood flow is said to reduce pain.

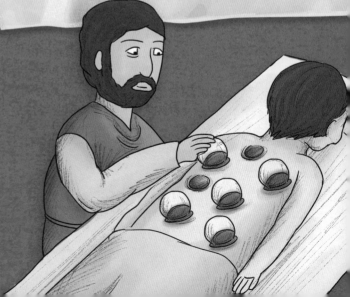

Blowing smoke up

When Europeans brought tobacco back from America in the 1500s, doctors thought it might help treat some ailments. But some doctors had a strange way of using it. They would light a pipe full of tobacco and use a long tube to blow the smoke up the patient's rear end! They called this a 'tobacco enema'.

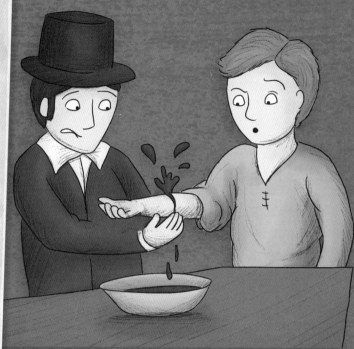

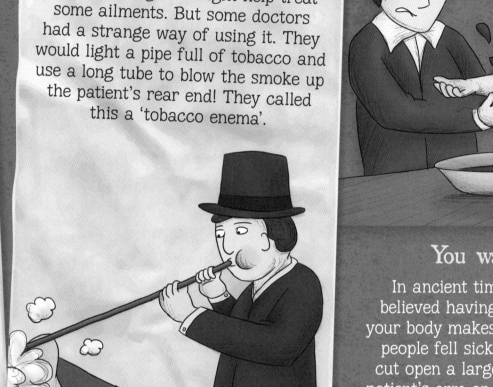

You want blood?

In ancient times, many doctors believed having too much blood in your body makes you ill. So whenever people fell sick, the doctors would cut open a large blood vessel in the patient's arm or neck to let out blood. Many died or became worse through loss of blood. But the practice went on until the mid-1800s.

Bloodsuckers

You didn't have to cut people to let out blood. Some doctors used leeches to suck it out instead. The great thing about leeches, they thought, is that they can stick on close to the diseased organ! Some doctors have recently suggested that leeches might be a good way of treating some ailments after all.

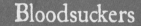

BARBERS AND QUACKS

In the past, there were all kinds of words used to describe doctors – not all of them nice! If you had a bad injury and maybe needed a leg cut off, you'd go to the barber surgeon. If you needed drugs, you could try an apothecary...

Quack pot

The 18th century was the heyday of 'quacks': people who tried to sell you their own brand of medicine – guaranteed to cure your problem! One notorious quack was American Dr Elisha Perkins (1741–1799). Perkins claimed he could cure rheumatism and pain by waving two metal rods or 'tractors' over you.

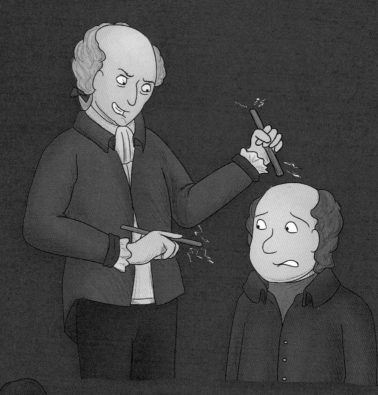

My legs grew back!

Some quacks made absurd promises. A 19th-century cartoon makes fun of the promise of miracle cures made by Morrison's vegetable pills. A man with two wooden legs claims his real legs have grown back, because he's taken Morrison's. The other man is not convinced!

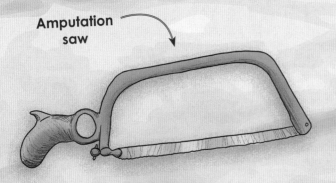
Amputation saw

Sawbones

In the past, if there was no way to treat a badly injured arm or leg, the only way to stop the wound going bad and killing you was to remove the wounded part with a saw. The men who did this were called 'sawbones'. Having your leg sawn off was unimaginably painful, since there were no anaesthetics back then.

Barber surgeons

In the Middle Ages, you didn't go to a doctor to have an injured arm or leg amputated – you went to the barber! Barbers were good with knives, so they could cut hair or limbs. They could also cut your arm to let out blood. That's why their symbol was a red and white pole, representing blood running down an arm.

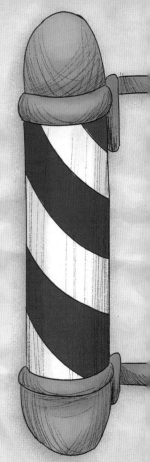

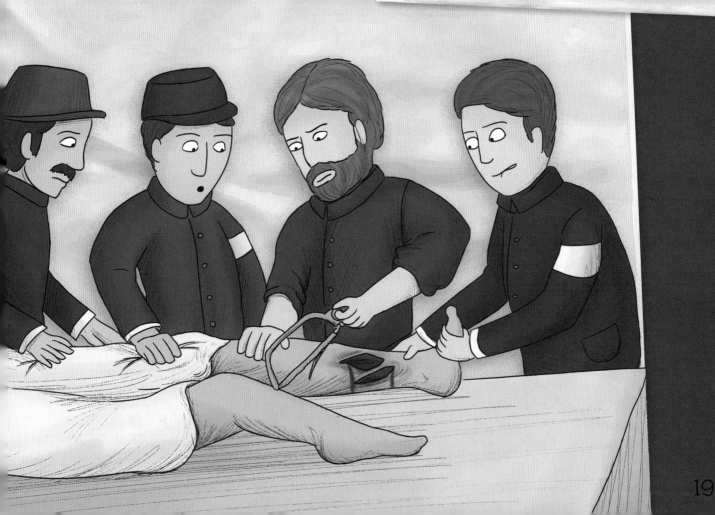

NEW BLOOD

If you lose lots of blood from an injury or during surgery, your life may be saved by an input of someone else's blood. This is called a 'transfusion'. We now take transfusions for granted, but in the past they could kill you.

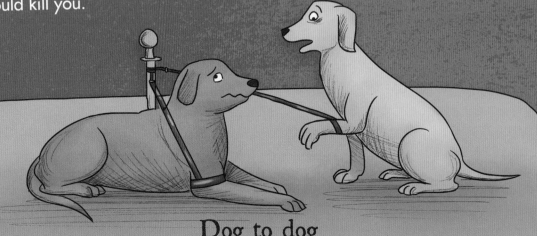

Dog to dog

The first sucessful transfusion was performed on two dogs in 1665 by English physician Richard Lower. He connected an artery in one dog with a vein in the other via a glass pipe. When he sliced an artery in the second dog so that it lost a lot of blood, it was kept alive by blood flowing from the first dog.

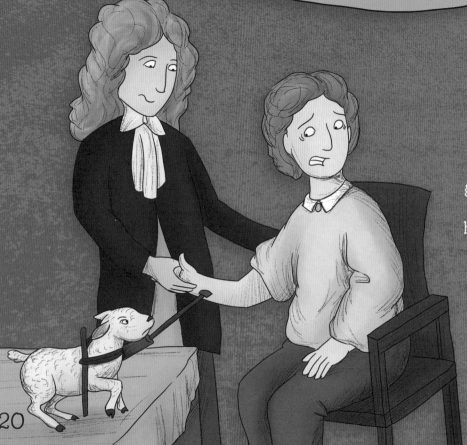

Bad blood

No one realised at the time that not all blood is the same. So in 1667, a doctor in Paris, Jean-Baptiste Denys, tried to give a man sheep's blood in the same way Lower had transfused two dogs. But the sheep's blood killed the man. Denys was tried for murder and transfusions were banned.

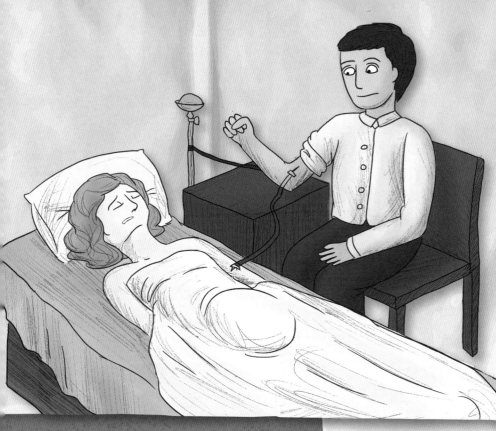

The first successful human transfusion

In the early 1800s, Dr James Blundell was appalled by how many women died from loss of blood during childbirth. So in 1818, he used a syringe to inject a mother who had lost a lot of blood with blood collected from her husband's arteries. The transfusion worked and the mother survived.

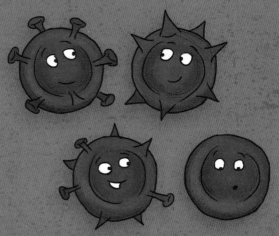

Blood types

Blundell's success was a lucky one-off, and most transfusions performed afterwards killed the patient. Then in 1900 Austrian-American doctor Karl Landsteiner (1868–1943) realised why. He believed that blood belonged to three different groups – A, B and O – and for a transfusion to work, the blood must be of the right kind.

Blood bank

The first transfusions were made by hooking the donor up directly to the patient. But then it was discovered that blood could be stored for several days in a refrigerator. In World War I, stores of blood called blood banks were set up, saving the lives of the countless wounded soldiers.

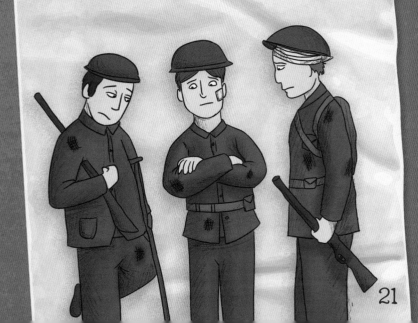

SICK HOSPITALS

It is said that the first proper hospitals appeared about 2,400 years ago and cared for the sick very well. But sometimes in the past, hospitals were horrible places as likely to kill you as cure you.

Holy hospitals!

Some of the first hospitals in Europe were in nunneries. But they could be terrible places where you might pray to get out alive. In the infamous Hôtel-Dieu in Paris in the 18th century, several people would be crammed into each bed, and patients with infectious diseases mixed with the mentally ill. Very few survived.

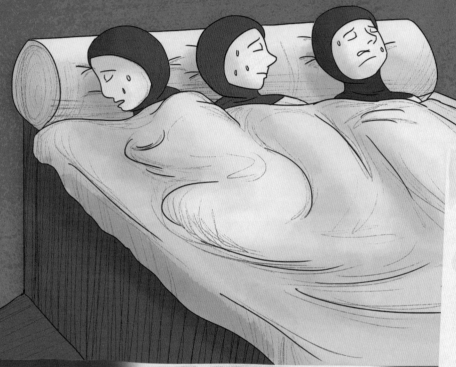

Lady with the lamp

Nurse Florence Nightingale was shocked by the crowded, dirty conditions in field hospitals for British soldiers wounded in the Crimean War in the 1850s. Her insistence on sanitary conditions, and taking close personal care of patients – even at night – helped change hospitals from places where people went to die to places of healing.

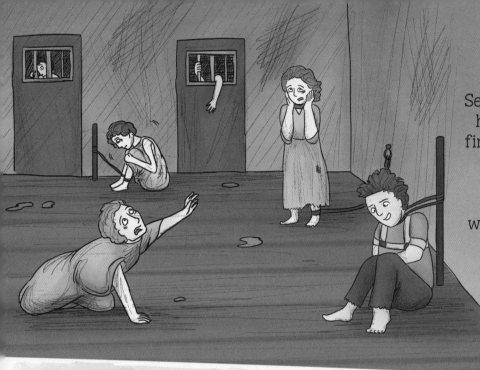

Bedlam!

Set up in 1247, the Bethlehem hospital in London was the first hospital for the mentally ill in England. But it was once a house of horrors, where distressed patients were chained up in appalling conditions. Their wailing was so horrific that the hospital's nickname, 'Bedlam', came to mean dreadful noise and chaos.

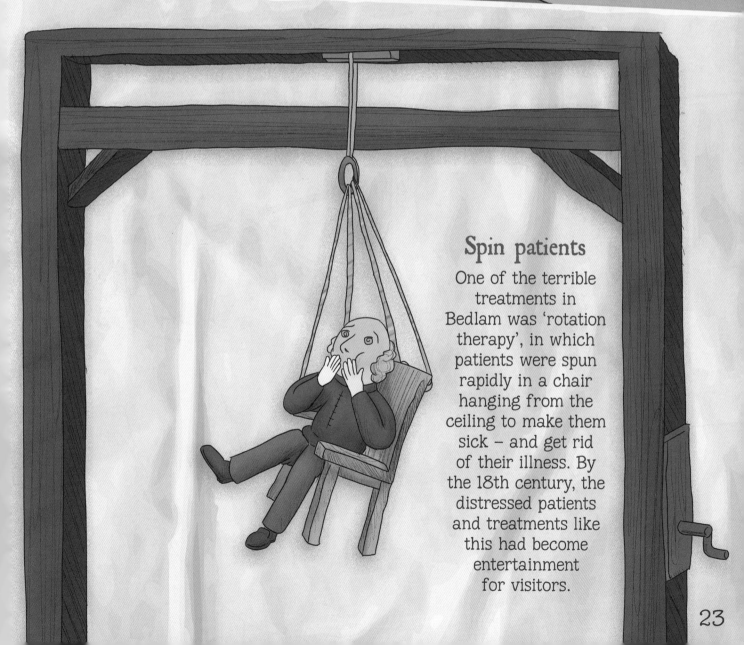

Spin patients

One of the terrible treatments in Bedlam was 'rotation therapy', in which patients were spun rapidly in a chair hanging from the ceiling to make them sick – and get rid of their illness. By the 18th century, the distressed patients and treatments like this had become entertainment for visitors.

23

TAKING THE PUSTULE

Your body can be protected against disease by deliberately infecting it with germs. The germs prime your body's defences, or 'immune system', to fight the disease. This is called 'inoculation'.

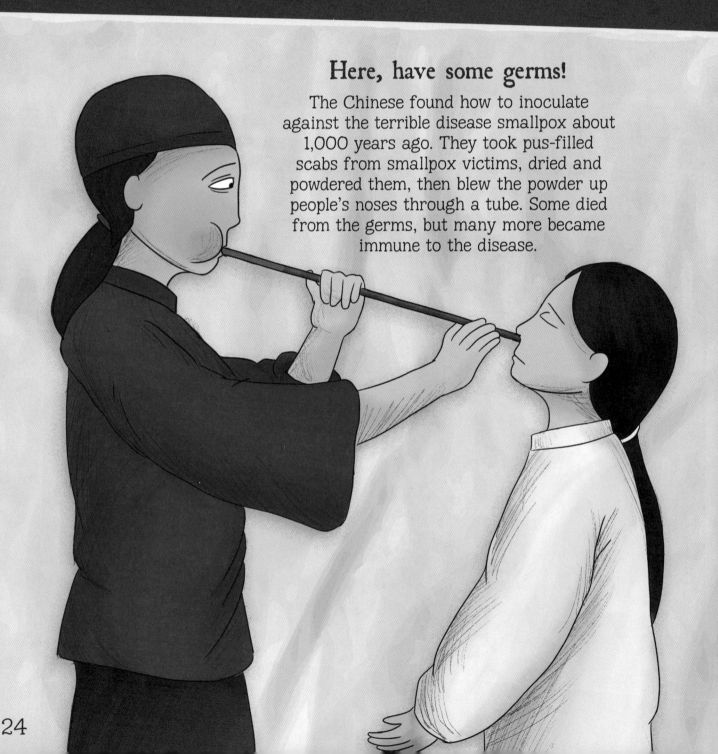

Here, have some germs!

The Chinese found how to inoculate against the terrible disease smallpox about 1,000 years ago. They took pus-filled scabs from smallpox victims, dried and powdered them, then blew the powder up people's noses through a tube. Some died from the germs, but many more became immune to the disease.

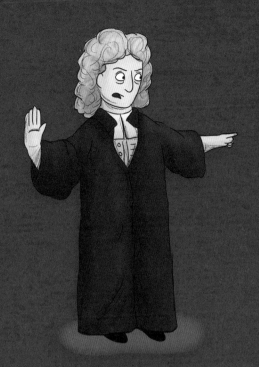

Beautiful milkmaids

In the 1700s, even those who survived smallpox were left badly scarred by the pustules. Yet milkmaids were famed for their flawless complexions. When they milked cows, it seems, they caught a mild form of the disease called cowpox and this made them immune to smallpox.

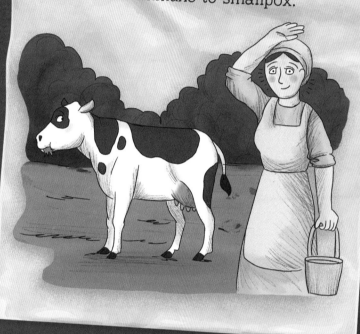

Inoculation in America

Smallpox once killed many Americans. But in 1706, Boston's Reverend Cotton Mather learnt about inoculation from his African slave. Later, in 1721, Mather persuaded local doctor Zabdiel Boylston to try inoculation in Boston. Many Bostonians objected that this was interfering with God's will, but the trials proved a success.

Vaccination

Inoculation with smallpox germs was dangerous. English doctor Edward Jenner wondered if cowpox germs might safely give the same protection. So in 1796, he injected cowpox pus into eight-year-old James Phipps. Luckily for James, it worked. Using mild forms of germs for inoculation is called 'vaccination'. By 1980, smallpox had been entirely eradicated from the world in this way.

CAN'T FEEL A THING

Without anaesthetics, major operations such as heart surgery would be impossible. Anaesthetics are chemicals that send you to sleep (general anaesthetic) or dull the pain in the affected area (local anaesthetic), while surgery is performed.

Sleepover

In 1847, Scottish doctor James Simpson had a party and tried out another anaesthetic, chloroform, with two of his doctor friends. It knocked all three of them out. Soon chloroform was being widely used for anaesthetising patients for operations. Then it was realised chloroform is slightly poisonous.

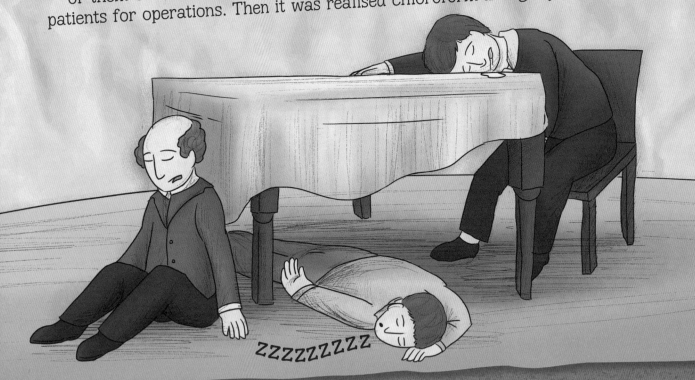

ZZZZZZZZ

It's a knockout

In Massachusetts in 1846, American dentist William Morton pulled a tooth out while his patient was fast asleep. This was the first public demonstration of an operation under general anaesthetic. The anaesthetic he used was a chemical called 'ether', which was warmed in a jar to create vapour that the patient breathed in.

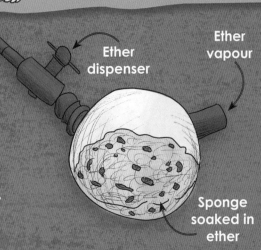

Ether dispenser

Ether vapour

Sponge soaked in ether

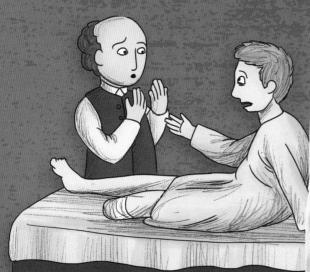

What a laugh!

In the 1830s, people went to demonstrations of the effects of nitrous oxide, known as 'laughing gas', because it makes you laugh and feel pain less. In 1844, dentist Horace Wells made patients breathe laughing gas from a pig's bladder and then painlessly pulled teeth out. But other dentists found patients cried out in pain midway through.

When are you going to begin?

Just a few months after Morton's tooth extraction, Scottish surgeon Robert Liston amputated a patient's leg while he was entirely unconscious from ether. The patient came round, entirely unaware the operation had been performed, asking Liston, 'When are you going to begin?'

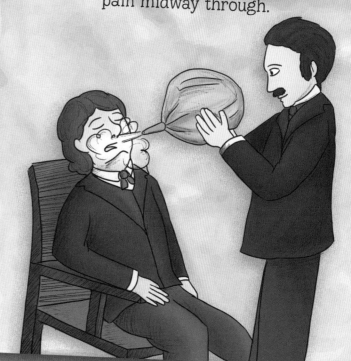

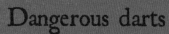

Dangerous darts

Some native South American people blow poison darts dipped in a plant extract called 'curare'. Curare paralyses victims so completely that they stop breathing and die. In the past, curare was tried as a general anaesthetic – until it was realised that although it made patients immobile, they could still feel the pain of an operation!

MEDICAL TIMES

Despite the sometimes odd treatments from the past, medical practice has made great progress through time. Here are some of the milestones.

About 420 BC
Science not magic

Greek doctor Hippocrates insisted that diseases have natural causes. He also insisted that doctors took an oath to treat patients properly. It is called the Hippocratic Oath, and doctors still take it today.

2600 BC

100 AD

About 2600 BC
First known doctor

It is said the first known doctor, whose name we know was Imhotep, lived in Ancient Egypt. He was also a priest and an engineer, and was worshipped as a god.

About 200 AD
Studying the body

Learning about the body from studying gladiators' wounds, Roman doctor Galen wrote a textbook that became the main guide for doctors for over 1,400 years.

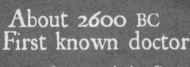

About 1000 BC Old herbalists

In India, the Ayurvedic system of herbal medicine dates back 3,000 years and is still practised today.

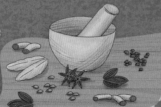

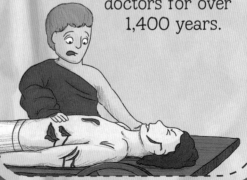

1818 New blood

Dr James Blundell made the first successful blood transfusion to save a woman from dying in childbirth. Now blood transfusions save hundreds of thousands of lives every year.

1967 Heart transplant

South African surgeon Christiaan Barnard performed the first human heart transplant, taking a healthy heart from someone who had recently died and swapping it for the failing heart of a patient.

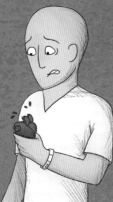

About 1030 Medical textbook

Muslim scholar Avicenna's *Canon of Medicine* became the standard medical textbook for the next 700 years.

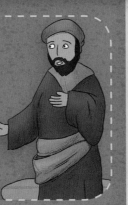

1900

1400

1540 Human anatomy

Italian Andreas Vesalius realised that to find out about human anatomy – what goes on inside the human body – he had to cut up real dead bodies.

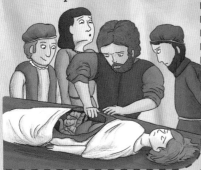

1846 Sleeping through it

American dentist William Morton publicly performed the first operation under general anaesthetic when he sent his patient to sleep with ether fumes while he pulled a tooth out.

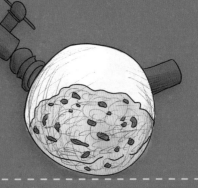

DOCTORS MAKE ME SICK!

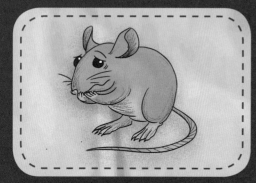

The Ancient Egyptians thought they could cure toothache by slitting open the belly of a mouse and laying its still-warm body on your gums. Ugh!

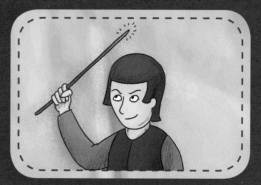

In the past, doctors stopped severe bleeding, perhaps after an amputation, by cauterising the wound – scorching it with red-hot metal or boiling tar. My goodness!

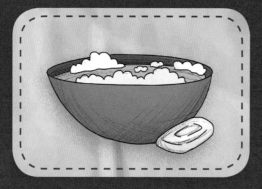

In 1738, the British parliament paid quack Joanna Stephens £5,000 for her bladder stone cure – but it was just soap and eggshells. Frothy!

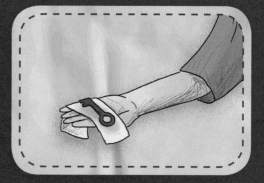

If you were bitten by a dog with rabies, a priest might scorch the bite with a red-hot key or nail, called St Hubert's Key. Surprisingly it could actually work if done soon after the bite, by killing the virus. Ouch!

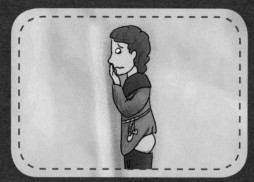

In the Middle Ages, if a doctor offered you a clyster to treat your illness, run. A clyster was a tube that he stuck up your bottom and then poured in hot water or pig's bile. Yuck!

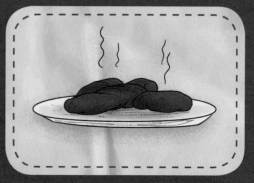

To cure a sore throat in the Middle Ages, a doctor might tell you to eat dog poo. No need to eat it wet – dried and mixed with honey was fine... Mmm!

GLOSSARY

Anaesthetic	A chemical that numbs pain or sends you to sleep
Bile	A dark green fluid made by the liver, and was related to a passionate, impulsive nature
Cupping	A medical treatment that involves applying heated cups to the skin to draw the blood to the surface
Diabetes	A disease in which there is too much sugar in the blood
Enema	The injection of fluid or gas into the bottom for medical purposes
Graft	To remove a piece of skin, bone etc from someone's body and put it onto or into another part of their body that has been damaged
Humour	One of four body fluids that old medical theory believed needed to be in balance to maintain good health
Immune system	The system by which your body protects itself against disease
Inoculation	The method of using germs to stimulate the immune system to guard against infection
Phlegm	The slimy stuff produced when you have a cold, and was linked to a shy, reserved nature
Transfusion	The process of putting blood from one person to another
Vaccination	The method of using dead or weakened germs to stimulate the body's immune system to guard against infection

Index

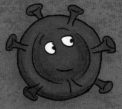
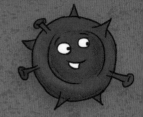
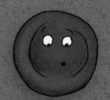

The Author

John Farndon is the author of many books on science, technology and nature, including the international best-sellers *Do Not Open* and *Do You Think You're Clever?* He has been shortlisted five times for the Royal Society's Young People's Book Prize.

The Illustrator

Venitia Dean grew up in Brighton, UK. She has loved drawing ever since she could hold a pencil. After receiving a digital drawing tablet for her 19th birthday she transferred to working digitally. She hasn't looked back since!

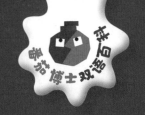

怪诞**医学史**

奇葩治疗术

约翰·法恩登〔英〕著

温妮莎·迪安〔英〕绘

罗来鸥 译

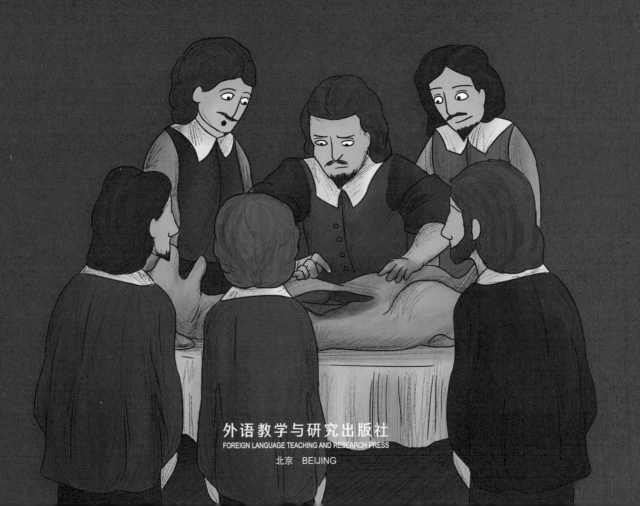

外语教学与研究出版社
FOREIGN LANGUAGE TEACHING AND RESEARCH PRESS

北京　BEIJING

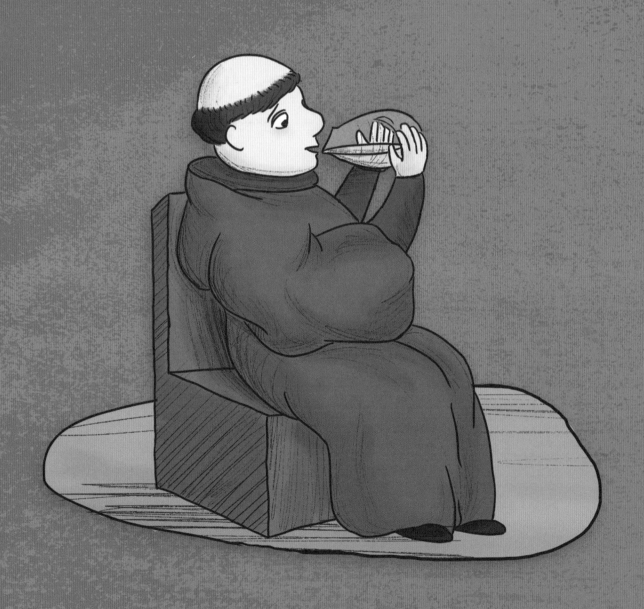

人类常被各类疾病所扰，寻医求药也从未间断。在过去，虽然大多数医生会想方设法治好病人，但他们的有些治疗方法令人匪夷所思，有些令人恶心，有些甚至相当危险。然而现代医学也正是起源于这些看似荒唐的实践。

● 将胳膊处的皮肤与鼻部缝合进行鼻部再造
● 第一次输血是狗对狗的输血
● 古代中国人将天花病人身上的脓液进行干燥、研磨处理，以防御天花
　　……

　　如果你胆子够大，可以继续往下看：拿剃头刀的理发师操起了手术刀，水蛭被放在病人身上吸血，盗尸者挖坟掘墓以供医生研究解剖学……但在这些惊悚画面背后，我们也欣喜地看到现代医学的伟大奇迹之一——人们发明了最早的、消除痛感的麻醉剂。

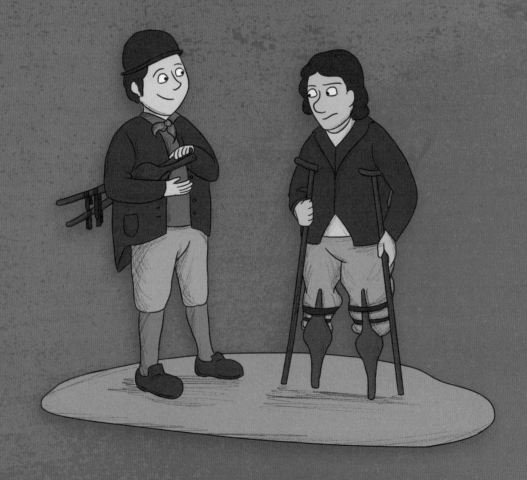

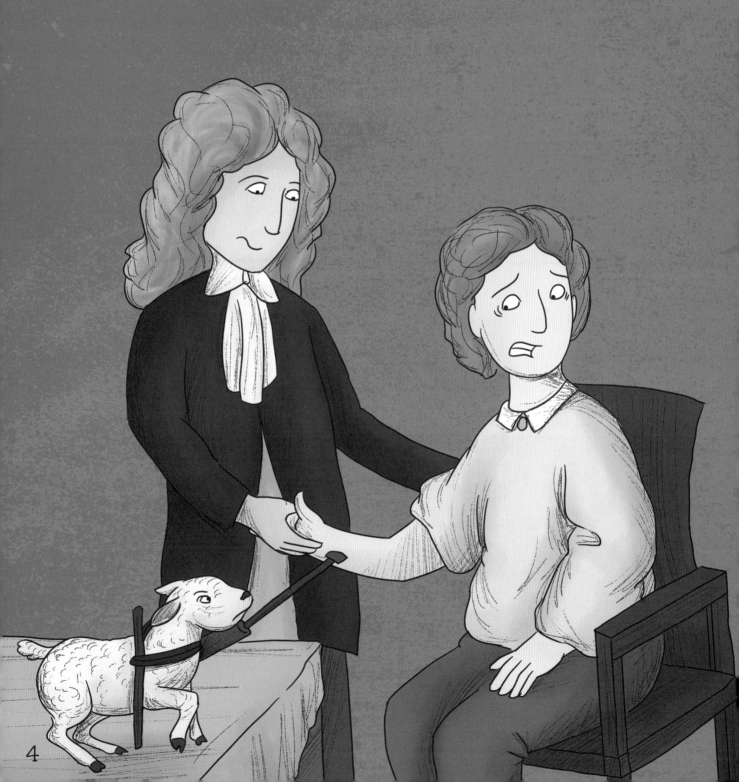

4

目录

写在前面

人类常被各类疾病所扰，寻医求药也从未间断。虽然大多数医生会想方设法治好病人，但在过去，他们的有些治疗方法令人匪夷所思，有些令人恶心，有些甚至相当危险。你能想象有医生愿意喝病人的尿液或者对着病人的肛门吹烟吗？要了解详情，就继续往下读吧……

我们需要更多的医生！

全球大约有6,900名卫生人员。世界卫生组织认为，在世界范围内，实际还存在400多万名卫生人员的需求缺口。

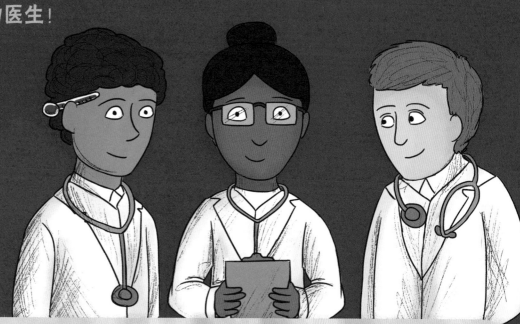

成为医生的条件：长期的专业训练

如果你想成为一名医生，就需要学习大量的知识和技能。要成为一名全科医生，平均要接受十年的培养与训练。一些专科医生需要经过长达16年的专业训练才能够胜任工作。

女扮男装的医生

早在古埃及时期就已经出现了女医生，但是她们通常不得不女扮男装才能获准行医。古希腊的昂格诺迪斯和生活在19世纪的英国军医詹姆斯·巴里（真名为玛格丽特·安·巴尔克利）就是她们中的代表。

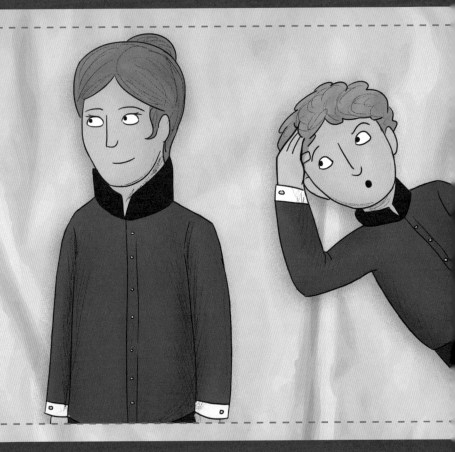

收入丰厚的职业

在美国，医生的收入通常都比较高。收入最高的科室之一是矫形外科，矫形外科医生医治骨头和肌肉，他们的年收入近为50万美金。

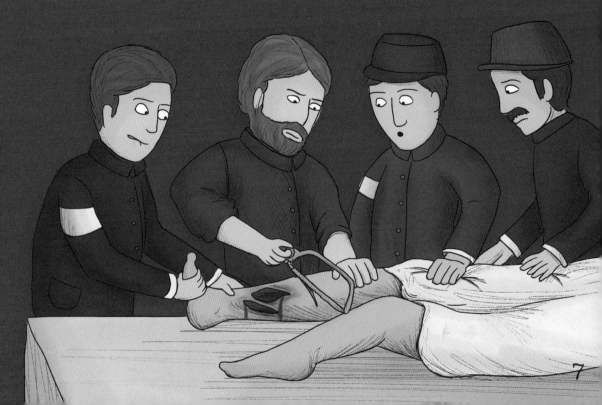

又切又钻的手术

如今的外科手术都是在病人麻醉的状态下，医生使用最新的高科技设备完成的，而最早的外科医生则是在病人躺在病床上痛苦惨叫的情形下进行开刀手术的。尽管这样很痛苦，但有时确实可能会救病人一命。

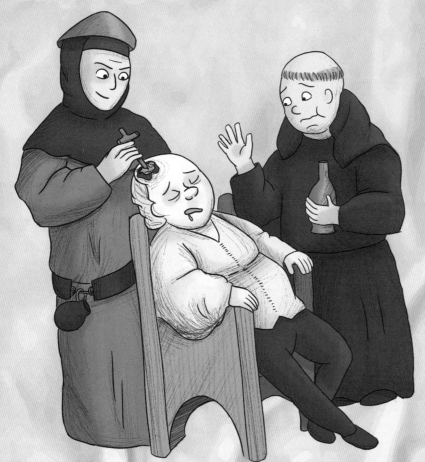

在头上钻洞

"环钻术"可以追溯到约7,000年前，它需要在人的颅骨上钻一个大洞。这听起来会让病人承受难以想象的痛苦并极其危险，但这种手术方法直至几百年前还在使用。没有人知道这样做的原因，或许是为了治疗痉挛，或许是要驱赶脑袋中的邪恶魔鬼。

缝合伤口

在至少6,000年前，人们就会用针和线将伤势严重的伤口缝合起来，他们使用的是骨针和动物筋腱或植物纤维制成的线。我们如今把这种处理方式称为"缝合术"。但在过去，或许人们只会用痛苦的叫声"啊……"来指代这种方法。

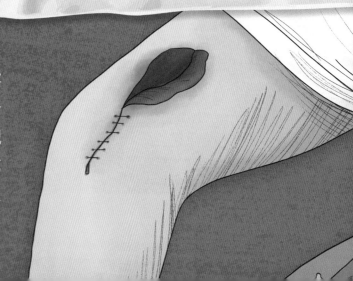

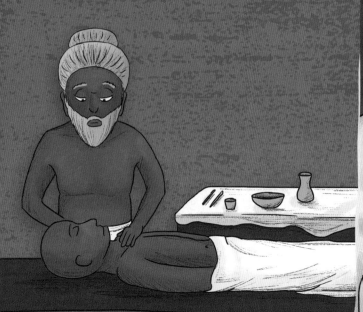

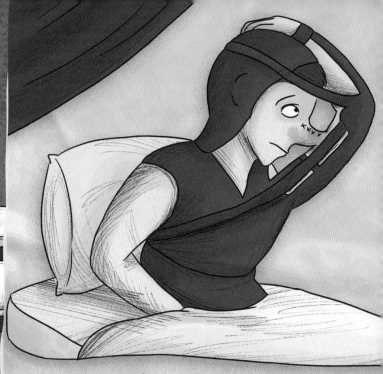

鼻子整形术之一

已知最早的整形外科医生之一是2,800年前生活在印度的苏许鲁塔。那时候，割掉鼻子是一种刑罚。于是苏许鲁塔发明了一种再造鼻子的方法。他从伤者脸上取一块皮肤，包在断鼻上，用缝线固定位置，直到和原来的部位严丝合缝，从而再造一个新鼻子。

鼻子整形术之二

在15世纪的意大利，如果有人在持剑决斗中丢了鼻子（好多人都是这样的），就会去加斯帕雷·塔利亚科齐医生那里求医。塔利亚科齐医生会通过移植伤者胳膊上的皮肤来再造一个鼻子。这意味着在长达数月的时间里，患者的胳膊和鼻子都会被缝到一起，而且这手术还不一定会成功。

一条黑腿，一条白腿

在三世纪的时候，君士坦丁堡的一个教堂执事腿部发生了感染。在他入梦后，本地圣徒科斯马斯和达米安对他说，不必担心。他们截掉了执事患病的那条腿，并从一位刚刚死去的人身上切下了一条腿，缝合在了执事断腿的位置上。但是那位死者是个黑人，于是，当这个执事醒来后，发现自己的双腿变成了一条黑腿和一条白腿。如果这个故事是真的，那么故事中的手术就是人类历史上第一例移植术……

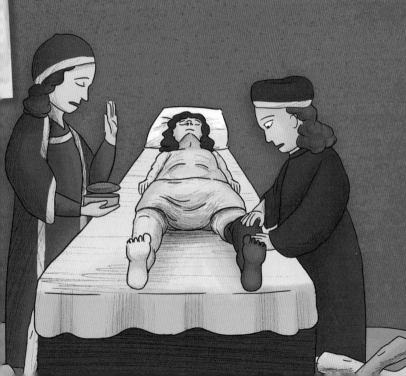

9

古代的医生

在史前时代，人们生病后依靠巫术和祖辈传下来的知识治病。而大部分现代医生则依靠科学知识诊病。据说，最早的专科医生出现在近5,000年前的古埃及时期。

拉伸器

古希腊医生希波克拉底（见右页图）发明了图中这个装置。在这个装置上，病人的胳膊和腿被套上绳子后，身体便被拉直固定在上面。这看起来很残忍，中世纪的刑具——肢刑架——就是受到了这个装置的影响。但是它的设计初衷是为了让断骨复位，现在的医院仍在使用类似的"牵引"装置来减轻受伤脊背所受的压力。

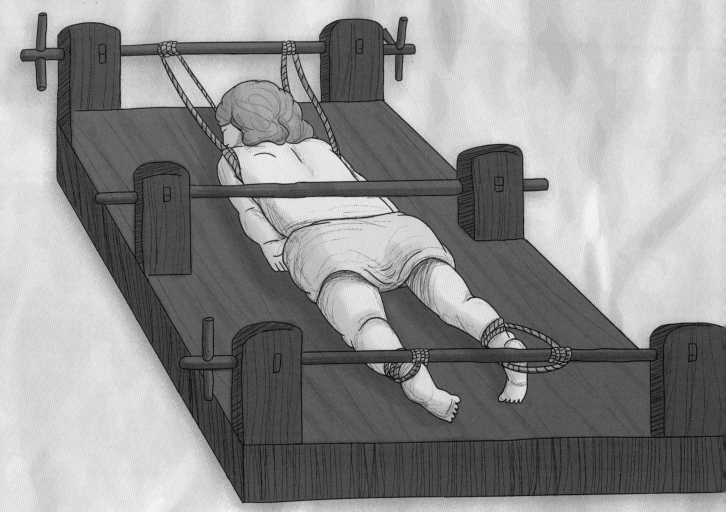

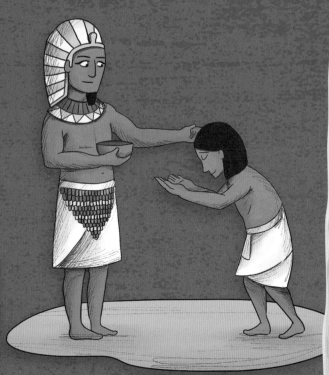

请不要用蛇！

大约2,500年前，希波克拉底生活在希腊科斯岛上。当时，古希腊的医生们经常试图用蛇的毒液来医治病人，结果经常把病人治死。希波克拉底知道这种做法是错误的——疾病不是神灵施予的惩罚，而是由自然因素导致的。他还提出医生有义务护理病人。

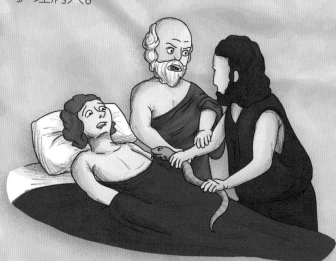

今天的医生仍会以全心全意救护病人为宗旨的希波克拉底誓言宣誓，这一誓言就是源于希波克拉底的从医理念。

"那就来个好墓吧！"

据说，史上第一位已知的医生是生活在大约4,600年前的古埃及医生伊姆霍特普，据说他能诊断和治疗约200种疾病，包括结核病和关节炎。他还懂解剖构造，或许对血液循环也有所了解。他还是一位建造金字塔的优秀工程师。所以，即便他不能治好你的病，也能给你修一个好坟墓！

"外伤治疗我拿手！"

盖伦（公元129—约216）是罗马帝国最著名的医生之一。他通过研究角斗士在格斗中留下的严重伤口，了解到了人体构造的真实模样。他所掌握的这些知识为其后1,400多年间的医学发展奠定了基础。盖伦曾自豪地说："我对医学的贡献堪比图拉真为罗马帝国建桥修路的贡献。"

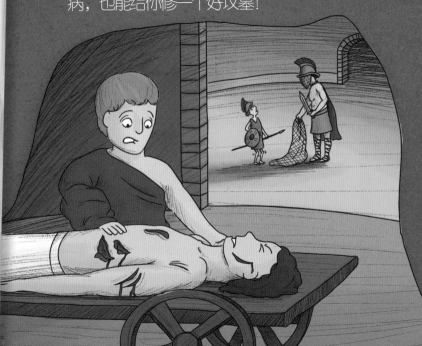

体液与性格特征

在古希腊、古罗马和中世纪的时候，医生认为人身体中有四种液体，叫"体液"。如果某种体液太多，人就会生病，而治疗的目的就是让各体液间恢复平衡。

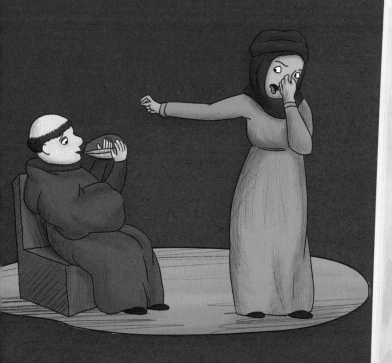

尿液中的"门道"

中世纪的一些医生认为他们可以通过病人的另一种液体——尿液——来判断病人身体出了什么毛病。他们不只是观察尿液的颜色，还会去闻，甚至去尝。想一想真是恶心啊！但是他们知道，尿液要是有甜味，病人就是患上了糖尿病。

每种体液分别对应病人可能会咳出的不同恶心液体。体液不仅会影响人的身体健康，还会影响人的性格。每种体液都对应不同的季节和天气类型。

第一种体液：黄胆汁

有时人可能把消化了一半的食物和这种黄色的胃液一起呕吐出来。黄胆汁与肝部的疾病有关；也和暴躁、易怒或者热情、冲动的个性特征联系在一起；还和夏季以及炎热、干燥的天气相关联。

第二种体液：血液

有时人可能会咯血或流鼻血。血液和心脏的疾病有关；也和活泼开朗、积极乐观、富有艺术气质的个性特征联系在一起；还和春季以及温热、潮湿的天气相关联。

第三种体液：黏液

黏液是人在感冒时咳出或打喷嚏时喷出的黏滑液体。黏液和腼腆、矜持、体贴和为他人着想的个性特征联系在一起；有时也和懒惰的性格联系在一起；还和冬季以及寒冷、潮湿的天气相关联。

第四种体液：黑胆汁

黑胆汁是人即使在空腹时也会吐出来的难闻液体。这种体液和脾的疾病有关；也常常和情绪多变、忧郁感伤又善于分析的个性特征联系在一起；还和秋季以及寒冷、干燥的天气相关联。

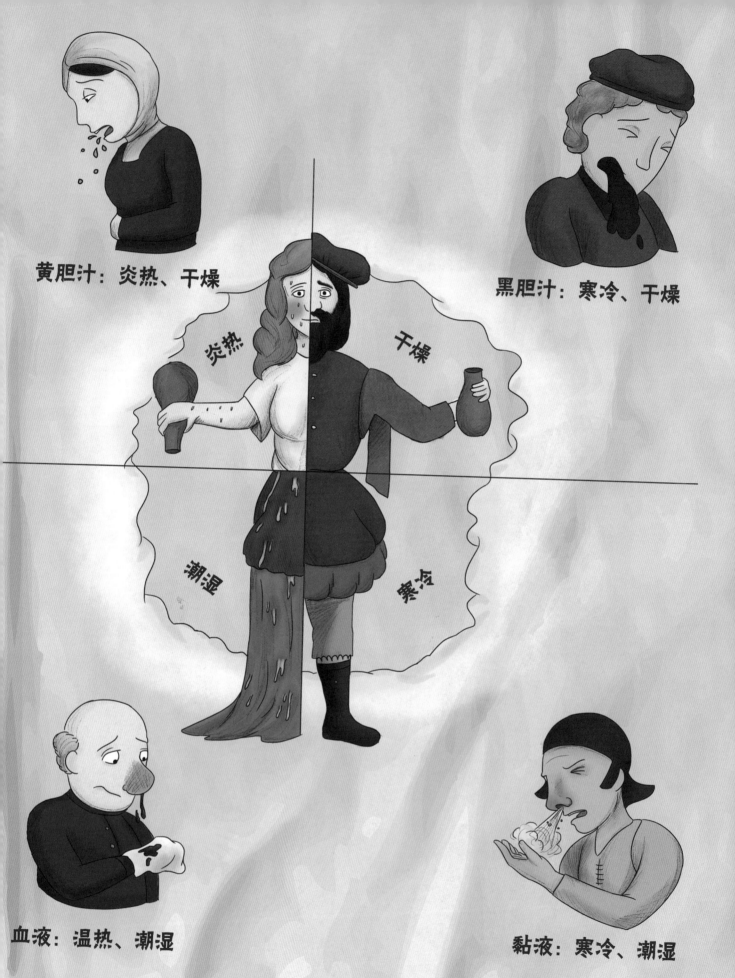

黄胆汁：炎热、干燥

黑胆汁：寒冷、干燥

炎热

干燥

潮湿

寒冷

血液：温热、潮湿

黏液：寒冷、潮湿

解剖学的发展

从16世纪起，人们认为了解人体内各个器官的位置（属解剖学范畴）以及它们的工作机理（属生理学范畴）或许能对医学发展有所助益。但是，这探索的过程可不那么美好！

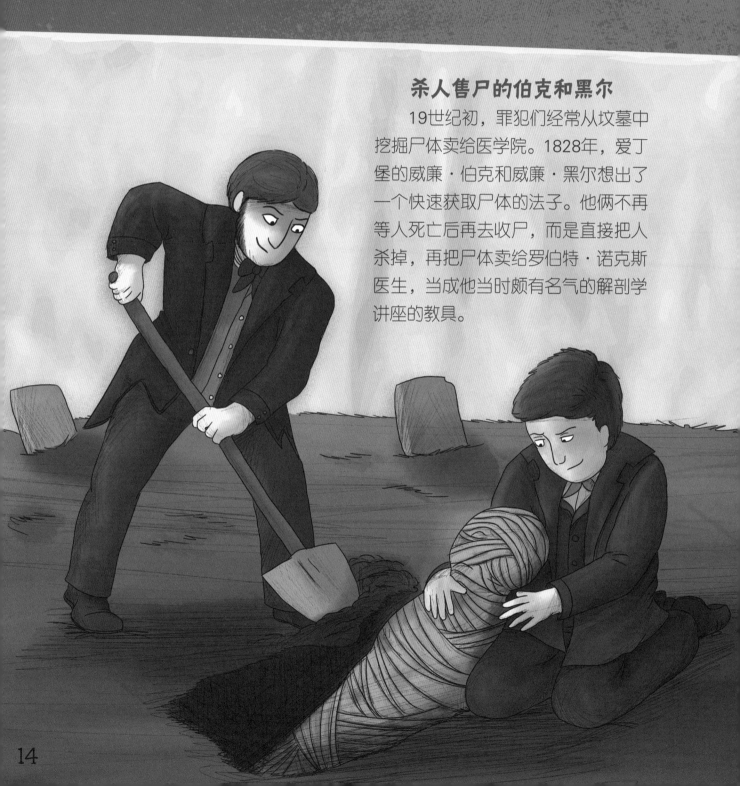

杀人售尸的伯克和黑尔

19世纪初，罪犯们经常从坟墓中挖掘尸体卖给医学院。1828年，爱丁堡的威廉·伯克和威廉·黑尔想出了一个快速获取尸体的法子。他俩不再等人死亡后再去收尸，而是直接把人杀掉，再把尸体卖给罗伯特·诺克斯医生，当成他当时颇有名气的解剖学讲座的教具。

"开膛破肚"的人体解剖

16世纪30年代，意大利医生安德烈亚斯·维萨留斯意识到，了解人体构造的唯一途径是将尸体剖开。他剖开尸体后，画出了详尽而准确的人体内部构造示意图。这种将尸体剖开的做法被称为"解剖"。1540年，维萨留斯在大批观众的围观下解剖了一名罪犯的尸体。

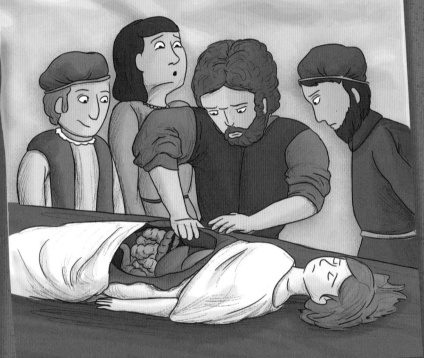

我说了只要半茶匙……

德裔瑞士籍医生帕拉切尔苏斯（1493—1541）提出了不同的疾病可以使用不同的药物对症治疗的观点。但他对毒药有着怪异的兴趣。当人们为此攻击他时，他回答说，所谓的毒药只有达到一定剂量时才称得上是毒药。他还曾在动物身上验证他的理论……

血液循环的证实

早在17世纪初，威廉·哈维就证实了血液并不是静止不动的，心脏会使血液在体内循环流动。这一发现是医学研究上的一大突破，但在今天看来，他当时的证实方式确实太过残忍。他把一只狗绑在桌子上，然后活生生地把它开膛破肚，以呈现这只狗的心脏搏动和血液流动情况。

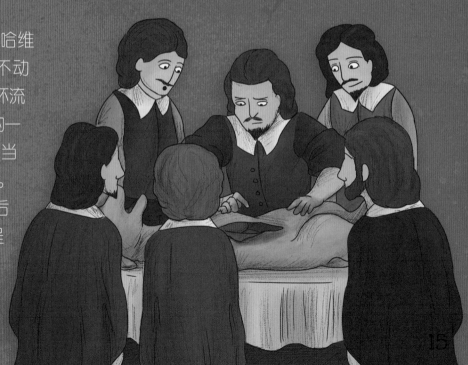

另类疗法也治病

下次如果你抱怨因为生病不得不吃药时，且想想，如果你生活在过去，生病的你可能会经历什么。医生或许会让你身上爬满吸血的蛭蝓，或许要割破你的皮肤放血，千奇百怪的疗法应有尽有。

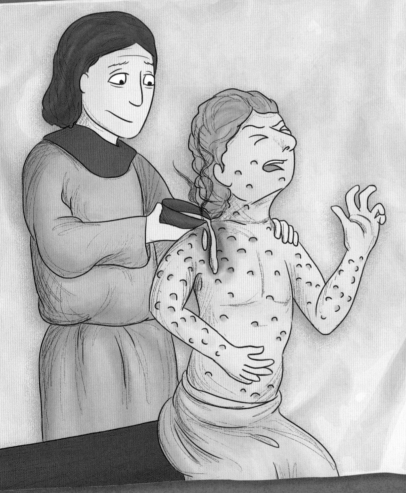

以毒攻毒的水银疗法

15世纪90年代，一种十分可怕的疾病——梅毒——开始在欧洲肆虐。梅毒的发病症状之一就是患者全身上下长满恐怖的脓疱。为了治疗这种疾病，医生会用匙舀取液态金属水银洒到患者的脓疱上，或者是让患者坐在充满水银蒸气的房间里熏蒸。但是水银本身有剧毒，会导致患者精神失常。

来个火罐？

拔火罐可以追溯到近5,000年前，直到今天仍然有人在使用这种疗法治病。拔火罐时，需要把罐子加热后牢牢扣到皮肤上。火罐的高温产生吸力，使拔罐处的皮肤充血。据说这样可以促进局部血液循环，缓解疼痛。

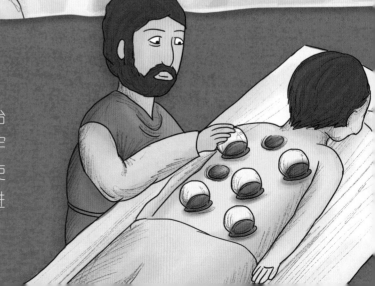

屁股"吸烟"能治病

16世纪，欧洲人从美洲带回了烟草，医生们认为烟草对治疗某些小病可能会有帮助，但一些医生发明了相当奇特的用法。他们点燃装满烟叶的烟斗，然后用一根长管子把烟斗里冒出的烟吹进病人的肛门。他们把这种治疗方法叫"烟灌肠"。

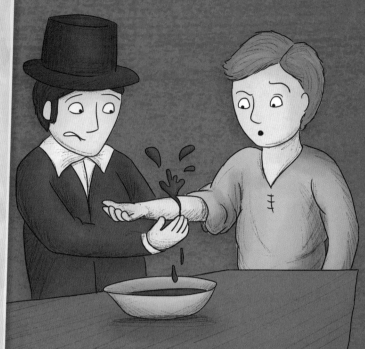

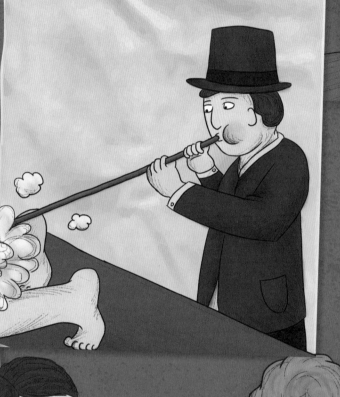

要血还是要命？

在古代，许多医生认为身体里的血液太多会引发疾病。因此每当人们生病时，医生都会把病人的胳膊或脖子上一根粗壮的血管切开，让血液流出来。许多病人因为失血而加重病情，甚至丢掉性命。但这种疗法一直使用至19世纪中叶。

吸血疗法也奏效

给病人放血也不一定要在他们身上划口子，一些医生会用水蛭把病人的血吸出来。他们认为用水蛭吸血的优势在于，它们可以吸附在有病变的器官附近。一些医生最近还提出，利用水蛭吸血或许算是治疗一些小病的好办法。

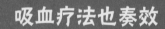

理发师和江湖医生

过去用来描述医生的词汇五花八门，但不是所有的词都是好词儿。如果你受了重伤，可能需要截去一条腿，那么你得去找"理发师医生"；如果需要吃药，你可以去找"配药师"……

江湖医生的"狗皮膏药"

18世纪是江湖医生们的"黄金时代"。这些二把刀医生会向病人兜售他们自家炮制的药物，并保证药到病除！美国人伊莱沙·珀金斯（1741—1799）就是一个臭名昭著的江湖医生，他声称自己只需在患者头上挥摆两个金属棒，或者叫"牵引器"，就可以治好风湿病、消除疼痛。

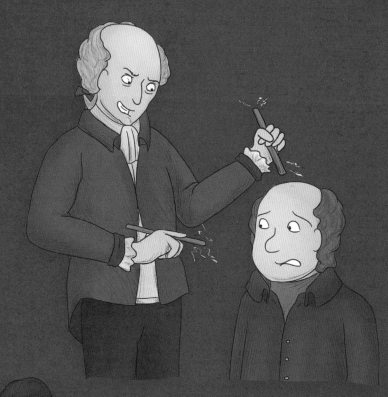

"我的腿长回来了！"

一些江湖医生还会胡乱夸口，许下一些荒唐的诺言。一幅19世纪的漫画就嘲讽了莫里森吹得天花乱坠的蔬菜药片。一个装着两条木腿的男子宣称，由于吃了莫里森的药片，他的真腿就长回来了，而他身边的男子认为他在胡说八道。

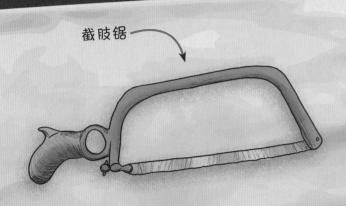

截肢锯

"锯骨医生"

在过去，如果一个人的手臂或腿上的伤势太重，没有办法医治，此时为了阻止病人伤势恶化而丧命的唯一办法，就是用锯子将受伤的肢体锯下来。实施此操作的人被称为"锯骨医生"。过去没有麻醉剂，因此接受锯腿手术的病人要承受难以想象的痛苦。

兼职做手术的理发师

如果在中世纪接受截肢手术，人们要找的不是医生，而是理发师！理发师能熟练地使用刀具，他们既能剪发也能截肢，还可以在病人的胳膊上割口子放血。因此理发店的标志曾是一根红白相间的柱子，代表血液顺着胳膊往下流。

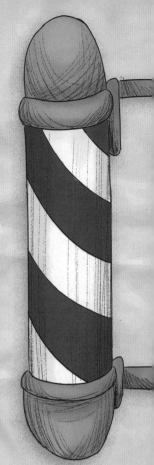

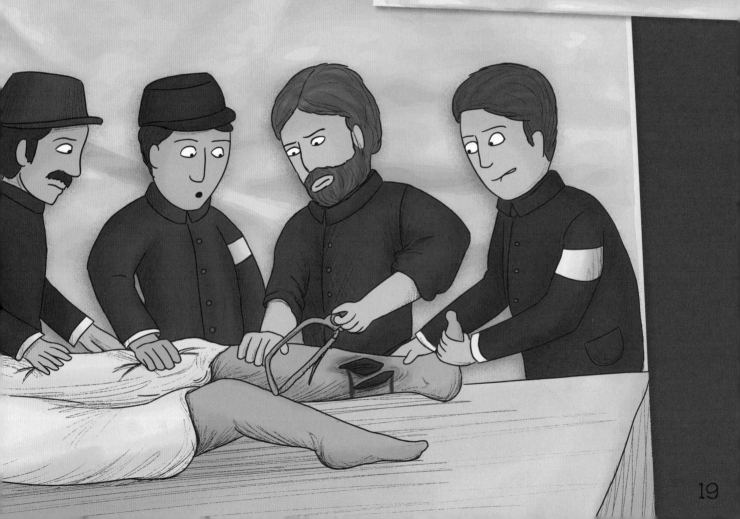

输血术发展史

如果你因受伤或手术而大量失血，输入他人的血液也许能够挽救你的生命，这就是我们通常所说的"输血"。如今，我们觉得输血是件小事，但是在过去，输血可能会让你丢掉性命。

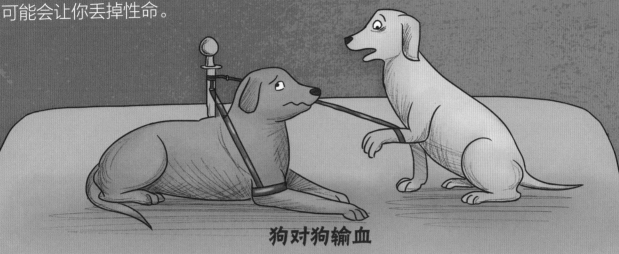

狗对狗输血

1665年，英格兰医生理查德·洛厄在两只狗之间实施了史上第一例成功的输血术。他用一根玻璃管将第一只狗的一根动脉和第二只狗的一根静脉连在一起。在他割破了第二只狗的一根动脉后，它便大量失血，但是依靠从第一只狗身上流淌过来的血液，第二只狗存活了下来。

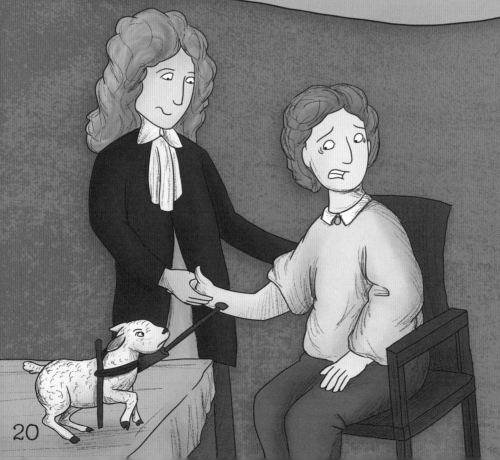

致命的血液

过去，人们还未认识到不是所有的血液都是一样的。1667年，巴黎的一位医生，让-巴普蒂斯特·德尼斯尝试仿照洛厄在两只狗之间输血的方法，给一个病人输羊血。然而，羊血导致了病人的死亡。法庭以谋杀罪审判了德尼斯，输血术也遭到了禁止。

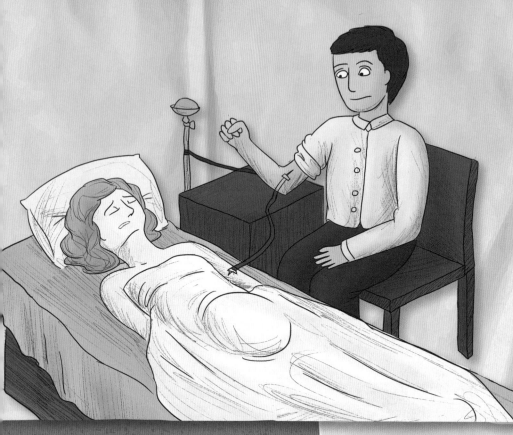

首次人对人输血成功！

19世纪初，许多女性因生产时失血过多而死亡，詹姆斯·布伦德尔医生对此深感震惊。1818年，一位产妇大量失血，他用注射器采集了产妇丈夫的动脉血，然后注射到了产妇体内。输血起了作用，产妇得救了。

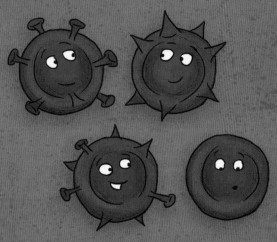

血型的发现

布伦德尔的输血操作只不过是侥幸成功，后来实施的大多数输血术都以患者不治身亡告终。1900年，奥地利裔美籍医生卡尔·兰德施泰纳（1868—1943）发现了其中的原因。他认为，血液分为三种类型：A型、B型和O型。要想输血成功，必须正确匹配血型。

建立血库

最早的输血是献血者直接把血液输给患者。但是人们后来发现，血液可以放在冰箱中储存若干天而不变质。第一次世界大战期间，人们建立了很多储存血液的血库，挽救了无数受伤军人的生命。

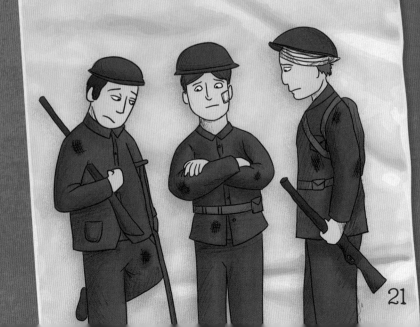

条件恶劣的早期医院

据说，约在2,400年前出现了第一批真正意义上的医院，病人在医院里可以得到很好的护理。但是，在历史上的某些时期，医院是一个可怕的地方，能让病人起死回生，也能让病人命丧黄泉。

令人"敬畏"的医院

欧洲一些早期的医院设在女修道院里。但是这些地方的条件可能很糟糕，病人要想活着出去，怕是只能祈求老天保佑了。在18世纪臭名昭著的巴黎主宫医院里，几个病人挤在同一张病床上，患了传染病的病人和精神病患者混在一起。在这种医院就医，很少有病人能够活下来。

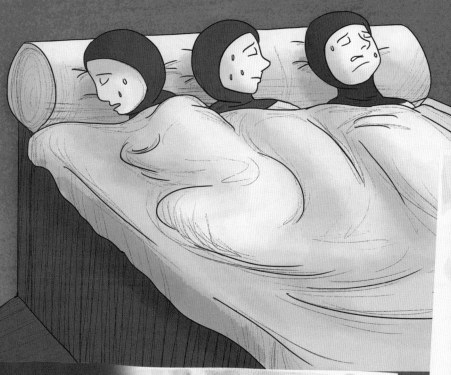

拯救病人的天使："提灯女神"

19世纪50年代，在克里米亚战争中，收治英国伤员的野战医院空间狭小、肮脏不堪，弗洛伦斯·南丁格尔护士对此深感震惊。她身体力行，坚持为伤员提供干净卫生的医疗环境，夜以继日、无微不至地护理病人。在她的努力下，医院不再是人们有进无出的鬼门关，而成了真正治病救人的地方。

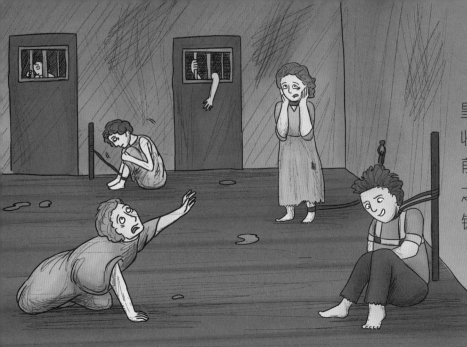

可怕的"疯人院"

建于1247年的伦敦伯利恒皇家医院是英格兰第一家专门收治精神病患者的医院。但在从前，它却是令人谈虎色变的恐怖之屋。在那里，精神病患者被用链子锁起来，遭受令人发指的对待。他们的哀嚎声令人毛骨悚然，医院因此得名"疯人院"——一个嘈杂混乱的人间地狱。

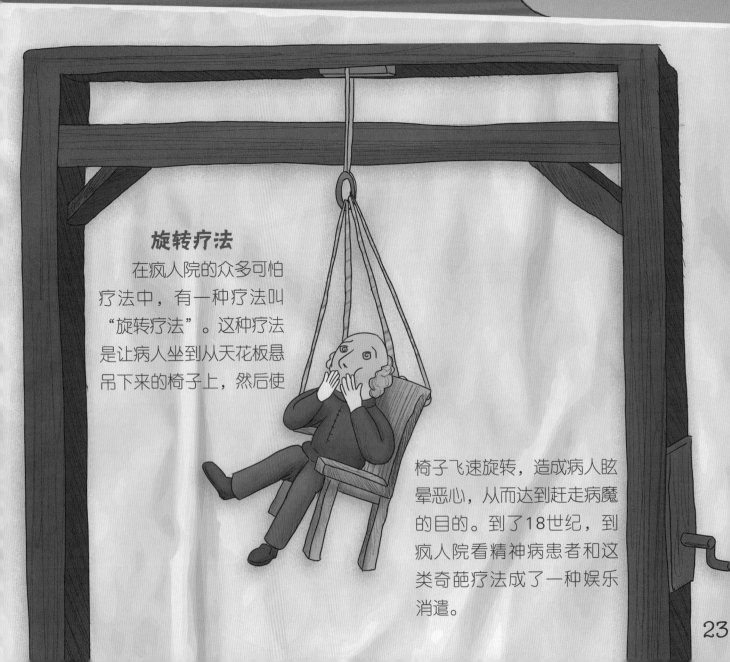

旋转疗法

在疯人院的众多可怕疗法中，有一种疗法叫"旋转疗法"。这种疗法是让病人坐到从天花板悬吊下来的椅子上，然后使椅子飞速旋转，造成病人眩晕恶心，从而达到赶走病魔的目的。到了18世纪，到疯人院看精神病患者和这类奇葩疗法成了一种娱乐消遣。

23

脓疱也是"护身符"

有意让身体感染病菌可以预防疾病，因为病菌会刺激身体中的防御系统产生应答以抵御疾病，这种防御系统也叫"免疫系统"，而这种治疗方法被称为"接种"。

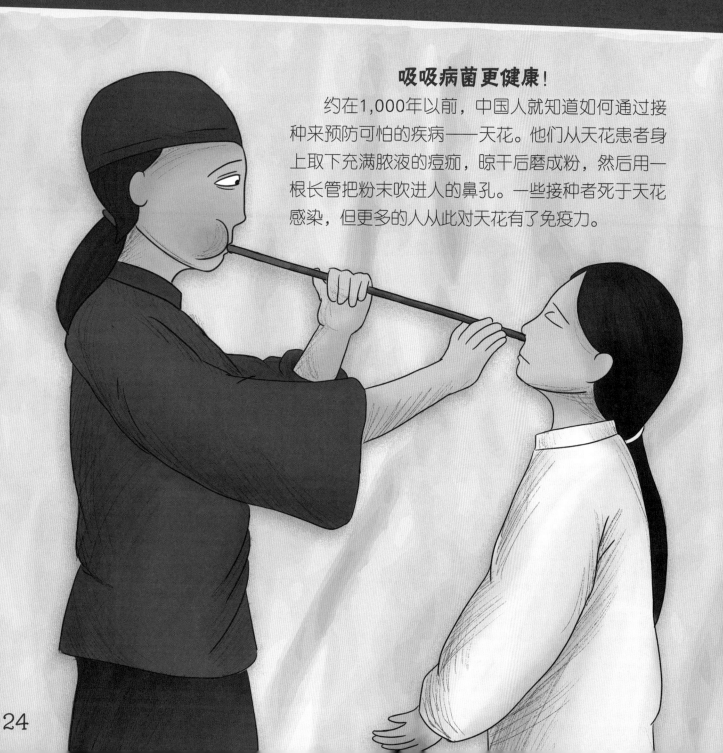

吸吸病菌更健康！

约在1,000年以前，中国人就知道如何通过接种来预防可怕的疾病——天花。他们从天花患者身上取下充满脓液的痘痂，晾干后磨成粉，然后用一根长管把粉末吹进人的鼻孔。一些接种者死于天花感染，但更多的人从此对天花有了免疫力。

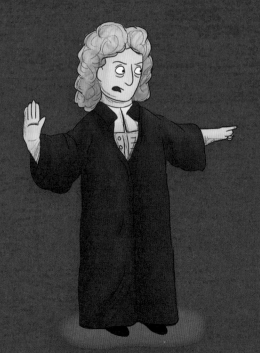

美丽的挤奶女工

18世纪，人们感染天花后，即使侥幸活下来，身上也会因脓疱留下累累疤痕。然而，挤奶女工的皮肤却是出了名的好。人们认为，她们在给牛挤奶时会染上一种类似天花，但症状较轻的疾病——牛痘，从而使她们对天花有了免疫力。

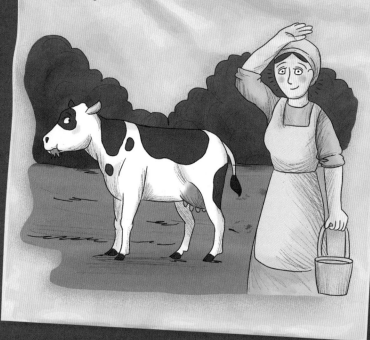

美国的接种试验

天花也曾导致很多美国人丧命。1706年，波士顿牧师科顿·马瑟从他的非洲奴隶那儿了解到了接种这种做法。1721年，马瑟说服了波士顿当地的医生扎布迪尔·博伊尔斯顿在波士顿尝试接种。许多波士顿人反对这种做法，他们认为这样做违背了上帝的意愿。但是试验证明接种是有效的。

疫苗接种

接种天花病毒很危险。英格兰医生爱德华·詹纳猜测，也许牛痘病毒能起到同样的预防效果，并且更安全。于是在1796年，他给八岁的詹姆斯·菲普斯注射了牛痘脓液。很幸运，牛痘病毒在詹姆斯身上起了作用。这种采用毒性较低的病菌进行接种的方法被称为"疫苗接种"。到1980年，人们通过这种方法已经在全世界彻底消灭了天花。

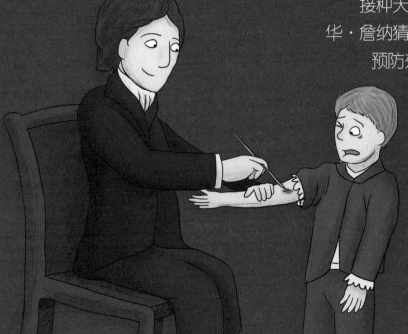

失去知觉为哪般

没有麻醉剂，像心脏手术这样的大手术是无法实现的。在实施外科手术时，麻醉剂是一种能让你昏睡过去（全身麻醉）或麻痹手术部位的痛感（局部麻醉）的化学品。

来睡一觉？

1847年，苏格兰医生詹姆斯·辛普森办了一个聚会。在聚会上，他和两个医生朋友尝试使用了一种麻醉剂——氯仿。用药后三个人都不省人事。很快，氯仿被广泛应用于手术时对病人的麻醉。但后来人们意识到氯仿有轻微毒性。

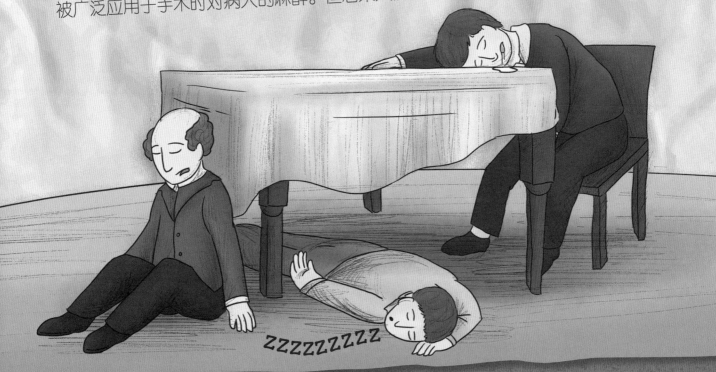

ZZZZZZZZZZZ

全麻手术

1846年，马萨诸塞州的美国牙医威廉·莫顿在病人昏睡状态下拔掉了他的一颗牙。这是在患者全身麻醉状态下实施的第一例公开的手术示范。他使用的麻醉剂是一种被称为"乙醚"的化学品，装有乙醚的罐子被加热后会挥发出乙醚蒸气，以供患者吸入。

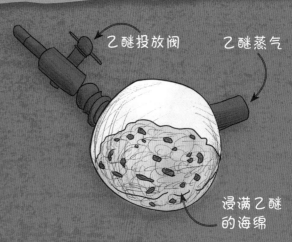

乙醚投放阀

乙醚蒸气

浸满乙醚的海绵

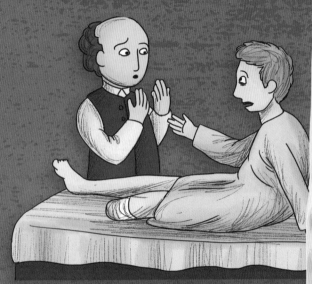

"您什么时候开始手术？"

就在莫顿成功实施全麻拔牙术后几个月，苏格兰外科医生罗伯特·利斯顿对一名患者使用乙醚麻醉剂，在患者完全失去意识后截掉了他的一条腿。患者醒过来后，完全不知道手术已经结束了，还问利斯顿："您什么时候开始手术？"

神奇的笑气

19世纪30年代，人们开始验证一氧化二氮的麻醉效果。一氧化二氮能让人发笑，减缓痛感，因此被称为"笑气"。1844年，牙医霍勒斯·韦尔斯让患者吸入充进猪膀胱里的笑气，在患者毫无痛感的情况下拔掉他们的牙齿。但是，其他牙医却遇到了患者在手术进行到中途就疼得大叫的情况。

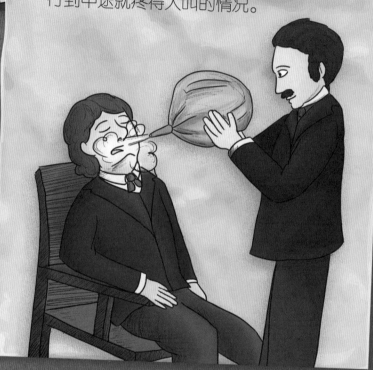

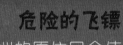

危险的飞镖

一些南美洲的原住民会使用吹箭筒射出毒镖，这种毒镖会浸在一种植物的提取物中，也叫"箭毒"。箭毒会使受害者全身麻痹，窒息身亡。过去人们曾经尝试把箭毒用作全身麻醉剂，但后来发现，虽然它能使病人不能动弹，但病人在手术过程中仍有痛感，于是就不再把它当成麻醉剂了。

回看医疗发展史

虽然过去的医学史上有一些稀奇古怪的治疗方法，但随着时间的推移，医疗手段已经取得了长足的发展。以下记录的是医疗发展史中一些具有里程碑意义的事件。

公元前2600年

公元100年

约公元前420年 确立医学的科学地位

希腊医生希波克拉底坚持认为人们生病是由自然因素导致的，他还坚持主张医生应该宣誓以全心全意救护病人。这就是著名的希波克拉底誓言，今天的医生仍然会用希波克拉底誓言宣誓。

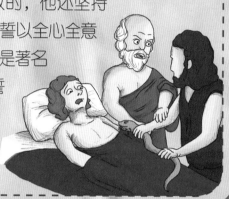

约公元前2600年 出现第一位已知的医生

据说，史上第一位已知的医生是生活在古埃及的伊姆霍特普。他同时也是祭司和工程师，人们把他当成神灵来敬奉。

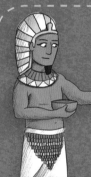

约公元200年 开始研究人体构造

罗马医生盖伦通过众多角斗士的伤口研究人体构造，并撰写了一部医学教科书，这部著作在问世后的1,400多年里一直是医学领域的重要指南。

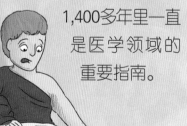

约公元前1000年 古老医学体系建立

印度的阿育吠陀草药医学体系历史悠久，可以追溯到3,000年前，且至今仍在沿用。

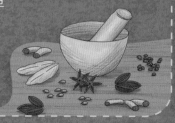

1818年 输血术成功

詹姆斯·布伦德尔医生成功实施了第一例人对人输血术，救活了一位在分娩时濒死的产妇。如今，输血每年能拯救数十万人的生命。

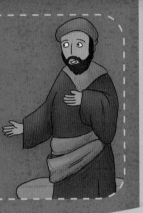

1967年 心脏移植术

南非外科医生克里斯蒂安·巴纳德实施了第一例人类心脏移植术。他从一个刚刚死去的人身上摘取了健康的心脏，移植给了一名心衰病人。

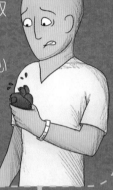

约1030年
权威医学教科书问世

穆斯林学者阿维森纳的《医典》成为问世后700年间医学界的权威教科书。

1900年

1400年

1540年 人体解剖构造

意大利医生安德烈亚斯·维萨留斯意识到要想了解人体的解剖构造，即人体内部的构造，必须解剖真正的尸体。

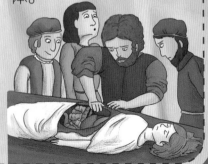

1846年 在睡眠中接受手术

美国牙医威廉·莫顿完成了第一例公开的全麻手术。他让患者吸入乙醚气体，使其昏睡过去，在此期间，他拔下了患者的一颗牙齿。

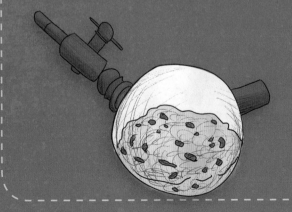

这些医生不靠谱！

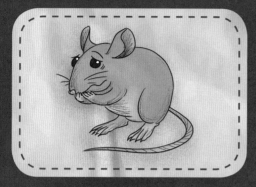

古埃及人认为，切开老鼠的肚子后，把它尚有体温的身体放在牙龈上可以治愈牙疼。呀！好恶心！

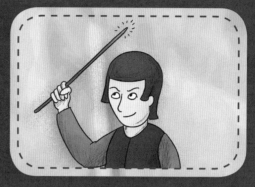

在过去，在做完截肢术之类的手术后，医生为止住大出血，会用烧红的金属或滚烫的柏油烧灼伤口。啊，好疼！

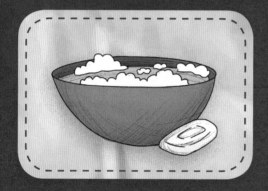

1738年，英国议会支付了5,000英镑购买江湖医生乔安娜·斯蒂芬森的膀胱结石药方，但药方中的配料不过是肥皂和蛋壳而已。不知道这些"药"制造了多少泡沫！

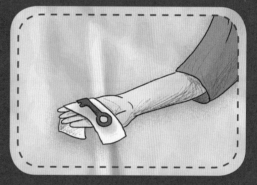

如果你被携带狂犬病毒的狗咬伤，牧师可能会用烧红的钥匙或者钉子烧灼伤口，这种钥匙或钉子就被美其名曰"圣休伯特的钥匙"。出人意料的是，如果在被咬伤后马上这么处理，还真能管用，因为这种烧灼可以杀死病毒。好疼！

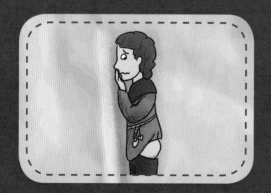

在中世纪，如果医生让你用灌肠法治病，赶紧跑！灌肠法是把一根管子插进你的肛门，然后向其灌入热水或猪的胆汁。太恶心了！

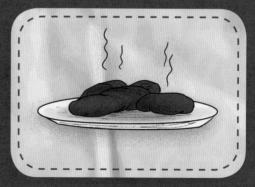

在中世纪，找医生治疗嗓子疼时，他可能会让你吃狗屎。但你不一定非得吃刚排出来的湿软狗屎，风干后就着蜂蜜吃就可以……无言以对！

术语表

拔火罐   一种将加热的杯罐扣压在皮肤上，以形成局部充血的疗法

胆汁   肝脏分泌的深绿色液体，旧时被认为和热情、易冲动的个性特征相关

灌肠法   将液体或气体从肛门注入体内的疗法

接种   接种病菌以刺激免疫系统产生应答，从而预防感染的防疫方法

麻醉剂   能够使人失去对疼痛的感知或让人昏睡的化学品

免疫系统   人体自身对抗疾病的系统

黏液   感冒时身体产生的黏滑液体，旧时被认为和腼腆、矜持的个性特征相关

输血   把一个人体内的血液注入另一个人体内的过程

糖尿病   一种因血糖水平过高而引发的疾病

体液   旧时医学理论认为人体中有四种需保持平衡以维持身体健康的液体

移植   将他人或自己身体其他部位的皮肤或骨头等移接到患处

疫苗接种   接种失去活性或活性减弱的病菌以刺激免疫系统产生应答，从而预防感染的防疫方法

索引

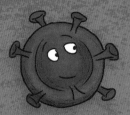
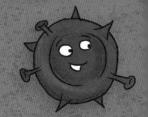
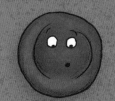

作者简介

　　约翰·法恩登是位多产的科普图书作家，作品涉及科学、技术和自然领域，包括全球畅销书《放我出去》和《你觉得自己聪明吗？》，并曾五次获得英国皇家学会青少年科学图书奖的提名。

绘者简介

　　温妮莎·迪安成长于英国布赖顿，从小时候能握住铅笔起就十分热爱绘画。她在19岁生日时收到了一个电子绘画板，便开始尝试电子绘画，从此在这条路上探索不止。